The Green Medicine Chest®
Healthy Treasures for the Whole Family

Also by Judith Boice, N.D., L.Ac.

At One With All Life: A Personal Journey in Gaian Communities

The Art of Daily Activism

Mother Earth: Through the Eyes of Women Photographers and Writers

The Pocket Guide to Naturopathic Medicine

"But My Doctor Never Told Me That!": Secrets for creating lifelong health

Menopause with Science and Soul: A guidebook for navigating the journey

The Green Medicine Chest®

Healthy Treasures for the Whole Family

By Judith Boice, N.D., L.Ac.

NEW YORK

The Green Medicine Chest®
By Judith Boice, N.D., L.Ac.

To contact Dr. Judith Boice for consultations or other information:
Web site: *www.drjudithboice.com*
E-mail: *drjudith@drjudithboice.com*

1% of the profits from this book are donated to support Green Medicine projects and oraganizations.

Note to reader: The information in this book is not intended as a substitute for medical counseling. Please do not attempt self-treatment of a medical problem without consulting a qualified health practitioner.

ISBN 978-1-61448-058-7 Paperback

ISBN 978-1-61448-059-4 eBook

Published by:

MORGAN JAMES PUBLISHING

The Entrepreneurial Publisher

5 Penn Plaza, 23rd Floor

New York City, New York 10001

(212) 655-5470 Office

(516) 908-4496 Fax

www.MorganJamesPublishing.com

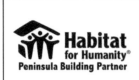

In an effort to support local communities, raise awareness and funds, Morgan James Publishing donates one percent of all book sales for the life of each book to Habitat for Humanity.

Get involved today, visit

www.HelpHabitatForHumanity.org.

To the Green World, the root of all medicine;
and to the Creator of All Things,
the ultimate source of healing.

Acknowledgements

Thank you to all of my teachers and mentors who have so abundantly and graciously shared their wisdom and knowledge: Kathleen Luiten, mystic and healer; AmyLee, woodland medicine woman; Dr. Jared Zeff, naturopathic physician and acupuncturist; James Kiji Watters, Shawandasse author, artist and medicine man; R.J. Stewart, author, musician and teacher; Ann Marie Holmes, author and Feng shui practitioner; Professor Hui Xian Chen, qigong instructor; Terri Applegate, qigong instructor and acupuncturist; the Green World and all of the Cousins; the Elements; the river of ancestors in whose wake I travel; and the Ancient Ones, the Masters.

Thanks to my cadre of editors, the best collection of grammar cops and spelling queens ever: Martha Boice (thanks, Mom!), Elizabeth Robinson and Catherine Rourke.

I am grateful to Micheal Reed Gach, founder of the Acupressure Institute of America, for generously granting permission to reproduce the point location drawings in the acupressure section.

Thanks to Missy Rogers for applying her mind, heart, hands and artistic eye to the creation of the cover art.

I am indebted to my beloved partner Jeff, for his love and support, and for his technical wizardry on the computer. Thanks also for watching the boys while I wrote (praise be, the house is still standing).

Thank you, Sebastian and Vincent, for providing the inspiration to send this knowledge into the world, for yours and future generations.

Table of Contents

Foreword

Selecting a name for one's book requires the same consciousness as naming a child. That moniker will forever remain the way both book and child are introduced to the world, complete with the public's accompanying expectations of it.

When my longtime friend, colleague and confidante Dr. Judith Boice deliberately determined the title for this most recent of her many books, *The Green Medicine Chest: Healthy Treasures for the Whole Family,* the innate value of its contents was guaranteed. The reader can trust this book by its title – it *is* a *treasure.* Over the past several decades Judith and I have intersected Medicine Paths, and each encounter has left us both stronger for the sharing. In Dr. Judith I found a "Sister of the Heart," a woman whose love of knowledge, healing and helping was built on both strong evidence (science) and a remarkable set of personal experiences. She is the someday-legend of the modern Medicine Woman, alive and walking amongst us today!

I do not use the term *Medicine Woman* lightly. While they are English words subject to numerous cultural interpretations, my use of the term here reflects a cadre of dedicated women who "give away" years of their lives in ultimate service to others via their pursuit of balance through wellness, healing, recovery and prevention of personal and planetary distress.

I was born into such a tradition of dedicated women. My aunties and grandmothers would gather, sometimes in ancient groves and other times in a house-bound auntie's apartment, always with the same goal. While ceremony and ritual would change, the content and connection followed true. Each woman would unfurl her blanket and set upon it many gifts and treasures.

Two of the medicine bundles would be opened for all to witness. The first bundle contained "the best medicine" each woman had discovered, developed and learned since the group's last circle. It would be thoroughly explained and then offered as a new tool to all in attendance who were drawn to accept that gift and its responsibility to use it wisely.

The second bundle held another equally potent gift: the same woman's vulnerability – that one illness, challenge or mystery that burdened her (personally or in her practice). It, too, was honored as a "Teacher, Tool and Gift" for those in the circle.

Each woman took her turn studying, pondering and drawing from her own vast pool of knowledge to offer insight, remedy or other incisive perception. All would return home richer for the treasures shared.

Dr. Judith has brought to you her own precious "treasures," gathered from far places, respected for their origins as much as their potency. And, as only Dr. Judith can do, she presents this medicine in a gently flowing river of easy-to-follow words.

I find most contemporary books on health to be collages of information pasted onto pages, with overlapping edges torn and glued onto layers of then-obscured truths. Dr. Judith's organizational excellence replaces all of those muddled manuscripts with a clear, concise book that is both a manual for well-being and the best kind of bedside reader one can pick up and enjoy, in or out of chapter sequence.

I actually read it both ways. First, a flip to whatever pages might open – what a treat! Dr. Judith's purposeful blend of her own experiences never upstages the topic. Those personal revelations connect us to her as being simultaneously real, identifiable and relatable to ourselves; they also read just a tad exotic by way of her globe-dancing medicinal adventures!

Next, I read it from beginning to end and have emerged with a rainbow of highlighted sections that now augment my own knowledge! (Thank you, Dr. Judith!)

True Confession: Growing up as I have, in a "woodland matriarchal medicine tradition," I tend to eschew others' attempts to mix traditions from many cultures, especially those indigenous to other environments. I can just hear my Gram now, defending her style of arranging her own furniture to a Feng shui promoter as being "the way it works here, *on this continent*" – meaning the way Gram liked it, was used to it, and the only way it all fit in the room.

In her defense, Gram would also be the first to say that all health requires flexibility – that we begin to die wherever we are rigid – in thought, habit, attitude, body and behavior. (Think of rigid arteries, for example.) Dr. Judith would make my Gram smile from the heart as she gently nudges us all into the flexibility required of us in these times.

Some "medicines," like some plants, do transplant well without disrupting the indigenous. And Dr. Judith found them. How blessed we are to have this

New Medicine Woman, Dr. Judith Boice, recover the paths for us to follow. I totally trust her knowledge, wisdom and integrity. I trust her with my life. Her book, *The Green Medicine Chest,* safely guides *you* to your own true treasure – a healthy family, a flexible self and natural peace of mind.

AMYLEE
Founder, Her Native Roots Herbals
November 2010

CHAPTER ONE

Green Medicine: The Quiet Revolution

When Steve first came to the clinic, his Environmental Illness (EI) symptoms were so severe he spent about 30-to-40 percent of his time in a semi-comatose state. A brilliant psychologist, Steve had periods of "brain fog" so intense he was unable to read or write. Some days he could barely speak. Almost weekly I made house calls to give Steve an acupuncture treatment for severe migraines that crippled him. He could not leave his reclining chair for days at a time.

At nine years old, Steve and his friends would chase after the truck spraying DDT along the edge of the park. The kids loved the feel of the cool spray on their summer sweaty skin. Nearly a decade passed before Steve began to experience the after-effects of these exposures. Bound for college on a full music scholarship, Steve suddenly lost all control of the muscles on his left side. Deeply frustrated, Steve couldn't even hold his percussion instruments, much less play them. Stymied about the cause of intense muscle contractions, Steve's doctor cut his neck muscles to relieve the spasms. Steve recovered from the mystery illness but faltered again in his early thirties, with a puzzling array of pain and fatigue symptoms.

When I met Steve, he had been disabled for nearly 30 years. He had received the very best, state-of-the-art conventional medical treatment available for his condition. Thankfully, this treatment had taught him how to manage his condition; none of the suggestions, however, had helped him regain his health. Slowly he had been declining, gradually losing function until his life had telescoped into a mobile home where he spent the majority of his time in a recliner chair.

Despite chronic pain and fatigue, Steve is one of the most tenacious, determined patients I have ever worked with. If he believes something will help, he dedicates himself to the process—100 percent. He has continued to struggle with an array of health issues, including two bouts of cancer. Over the last eight years, using many of the treatments you will discover in this book, Steve has gradually climbed from losing days at a time to "chronic fatigue fog," as he describes it, to being alert all of his waking hours—reading books and magazines and leaving his house for errands as well as a few longer trips.

THE QUIET REVOLUTION

If you are holding this book, you are part of a growing majority who are interested in taking control of their lives and *building* greater levels of health. Like Steve, you are part of a quiet revolution—the "greening" of health care.

In recent years, people have voted for natural health care by investing twice as much of their increasingly scarce dollars in natural supplements. You are on the crest of a wave, a growing swell of people who are choosing to take health care, true health-building, into their own hands.

Is your medicine chest filled with supplements you are not quite sure of how to use, OR are you ready to step into even greater levels of health?

I am offering you my hard-won knowledge from nearly 40 years of working with natural medicines. I did not always think this way about health. My childhood was mostly lost to illness—a few serious conditions but primarily chronic, low-grade sickness that sapped the joy out of living. I was a "victim" of these maladies. I "caught" colds and "came down" with other illnesses. Like most people, I felt helpless as my body passively succumbed to these infections.

What allowed me to slowly reclaim some semblance of control over my physical body? Food offered the first opening. When I was 13, a doctor tested me for food allergies. After removing these allergens from my diet a three-month bout of bronchitis cleared in two weeks.

The other kids at school couldn't believe I was crunching rice cakes with almond butter while they wolfed down pepperoni pizza with extra cheese. I had had enough of feeling victimized by illness. If something as simple as changing my diet could avert sickness, I was delighted to make the "sacrifice."

So, *taking away* the offending substances became my first approach—beginning with food and then moving on to eliminating pharmaceutical drugs and noxious chemicals. Gratefully, I made progress as I removed straws from the camel's back.

I continued "avoidance" therapy for about a decade, until I began to learn the fundamentals of rebuilding health. Slowly, I discovered that taking straws off the camel's back might not provide enough additional energy to rebuild health. The worn beast of burden—in this, case my body—might need additional input and NOT just less output to rejuvenate.

Thus, I entered the world of botanicals, long-distance running and ceremony. I explored emotions and thoughts and learned how these powerful experiences shape the physical body. I was convinced that every illness had not just a physical but also a mental, emotional and/or spiritual basis.

Several more years passed before I studied with a gifted philosopher of natural medicine, Jared Zeff, N.D., LAc. After completing naturopathic medical school in the 1970s, Dr. Zeff had been disillusioned with his results in working with patients. He was contemplating entering conventional medical school when he met Harold Dick, N.D., a naturopathic physician who had been practicing for more than 40 years. Dr. Dick worked primarily with dietary changes and constitutional hydrotherapy treatments, a particular therapy that deeply rebuilds both immune and digestive function. These deceptively simple treatments wrought miraculous changes in Dr. Dick's patients.

Dr. Zeff apprenticed himself to Dr. Dick, visiting his clinic several times over the next couple of years. Dr. Zeff also studied ancient medical texts, hoping to glean the secrets of these masters. He read Hippocrates, searching for the keys to vitality and health.

"I was frustrated," recalls Dr. Zeff. "Hippocrates would say, 'I saw so-and-so and they had these symptoms. They were eating this diet. I told them to eat this and this. Then I saw so-and-so.' Hippocrates described case after case, always noting the patient's diet and then what he told them to eat.

"I was after the secrets of medicine, so I kept reading case after case. Finally, it dawned on me. This WAS the secret. What we eat *is* the foundation of our health. There it was, right in front of me. The secret was so obvious I couldn't see it."

From his experience and study, Dr. Zeff created or, in truth, re-created a model of developing disease *and restoring health* (see "Paradigm of Health and Disease" below). Like most depictions of truth, his model is deceptively simple.

With this working model of disease and health, I entered a new realm of true health promotion, not just symptom eradication. The previous two decades of study, collecting a disparate assortment of treatments, coalesced into a unified whole with this viewpoint.

So many people, and myself included, enter "natural health care" by simply substituting more "natural" substances for pharmaceutical or over-the-counter drugs. Initially, I still operated in the same mental framework I call "taking this for that"—zinc for sore throats, comfrey for wound healing and Echinacea for colds. I did not have a framework of using natural therapies to rebuild health but only to eradicate symptoms.

My quiet revolution had begun with the "greening" of my medicine chest and my life. Instead of relying on pharmaceuticals synthesized from petrochemicals, my medicine cabinet was now filled with the bounty of this land—herbs, clay, nutrients, essential oils and flower essences. I could use these extraordinary tools not only to reduce symptoms, but also to create the energized body I had always wanted.

Thank goodness pharmaceutical drugs are there for emergencies—that's what they've always been intended for. Prescription medications were never meant to restore health, only to treat disease.

So open the "green" treasure chest; swing wide the door. The land and all of its gifts are the most effective, most sustainable form of medicine to rebuild health.

THE ROOTS OF GREEN MEDICINE

This Green Medicine guide is intended to help you regain the wisdom that is available to each of us, if we have the eyes to see and the ears to listen. This ancient knowledge lives amidst us, literally in the soil at our feet. We need only learn how to listen respectfully to the land and its inhabitants for direction in how both to nurture and receive the gifts around us.

One of the most common plant allies in North America is plantain. This "lowly" plant has extraordinary healing powers. Likely, you have an abundance of this "weed" in your yard. Plantain is a vulnerary, meaning it soothes and lubricates; it is high in nutrients; and the seeds are a wonderful bulking agent and intestinal lubricant for constipation.

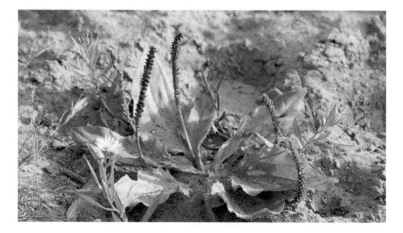

Julia Adamson

With book in hand, walk outside and see if you can locate plantain. Unless you live in the desert Southwest, or in an area with no irrigation, you likely have plantain in your yard.

When you find the plantain, bend down and look closely at it. Notice where the plant is growing—why here? Is there seepage from an irrigation ditch or a brown patch in the grass after last summer's drought? Notice that this plant thrives without need of invitation or cultivation. Plantain is a colonizer of damaged land, bringing gifts of healing and rejuvenation with it.

Bend down and stroke the leaves. Offer something of yourself before you pick a leaf and taste it. I was trained to offer one of my hairs—something that causes a bit of pain— to remind me that the plant experiences pain, too, when I pluck the leaves. I pull one of the hairs from my head and lay it next to the plant, letting it know I want to harvest one of its leaves. I aim to gather one leaf from several plants, rather than decimating a single plant. With each leaf, I say "thank you," either within my heart or out loud, as I harvest the plants' treasures.

Eating something from the earth around you attunes you to the land in that place. Many medicine people will eat a leaf from a tree, bush, or other plant before they begin to "work" in a particular area. As you ingest plants from the surrounding landscape, you literally begin to build your body from the elements where you live—minerals from the soil; water from the rain, the local river and the aquifer beneath you; air from your region; and the fire of the sun, as it slants at the particular angle where you live.

This attunement to the earth where you live is a vital part of learning "deep listening." This art of deep connection with the land offers many rewards. You begin to hear the voices of the earth's inhabitants around you. Without this primary skill of listening, all of the information in this book will literally fall on deaf ears. With this skill, you will hear and sense all of the subtle nuances of these green allies who are ready and very willing to share their healing knowledge.

Before you eat the plantain leaf, take a few moments to sit with it in your hand. You can also sit with the plant before you harvest a leaf. Sense your heart and breathe the essence of this plant right into the center of your chest. Relax and breathe for a few minutes, focusing on your heartbeat. Notice any thoughts or feelings that arise as you sit with the plant.

See Chapter 2 for more information about deep listening. For a recorded version of this exercise, visit: *http://www.drjudithboice.com/plantmeditation.html*

CLASSICAL MEDICINE

Green Medicine draws its strength from a group of medical approaches that I call "Classical Medicine." These are highly developed forms of healing that long pre-date our current conventional medical system. When people talk about going to see their "traditional" medical practitioner, I chuckle. A form of medicine developed over the last century is hardly a "traditional" medicine; most of the schools and systems of medicine we will be addressing have roots that go back thousands of years.

In Chapter Two we will explore Classical Medicine principles in depth—the roots that nourish the tree of health and wholeness. Common to all of these systems of medicine is the understanding that the body is an organism, a highly refined, interactive system that has the ability to regenerate and restore itself. In contrast, the conventional medical system views the body as a machine with interchangeable parts that can be replaced or "fixed."

If you are interested in a discussion of this fundamental difference, or "split" in medical approaches, read *Divided Legacy: A History of the Schism in Medical Thought Volume IV* by Harris Coulter (North Atlantic Books, 1994). The basic message is that the medical worlds diverged when the current conventional medical system veered to viewing the body as a machine rather than an organism.

This shift gained momentum with the Industrial Revolution. Up to that time, in the 18th century, humans had always lived within the Earth's "carrying capacity," living in a way that was sustainable for the Earth. Our lives, our very survival, were allied with the health of the Earth.

In order to fuel the Industrial Revolution, our thinking had to shift. We had to see the Earth as a non-living resource, a mere Lego™ toy for our use and pleasure. The sheer volume of resources needed to fuel our culture of over-consumption meant we had to leave behind the sustainable agricultural methods developed over many millennia.

Our body is our own microcosm of the Earth. Divorcing ourselves from the sustainable cycles of Earth meant that we also divorced ourselves from our physical bodies. My physical earth and the planet Earth are one and the same.

Conventional medicine as it is practiced today is the first medical system developed after the Industrial Revolution. This system parallels the factory model of production—we mass-produce medicine and expect each person to react the same way to these substances. We place our health on assembly lines, adhering to the theories of standardization that fueled the early production line factories. Henry Ford mastered this particular form of factory production to mass-produce cars for a culture eager for easy, fast transportation.

Similarly, we are taught that our bodies should respond quickly and easily to the mass-produced medicines developed by the pharmaceutical industry. Strangely, though, many of our bodies do not respond well to this factory-model of treatment. We currently are reaching the limits of this approach. We are learning the very real, very complex truth that our bodies vary—no two are exactly alike.

Comb through your yard, look at the plantain leaves, and you will find the same is true of the plantain. Even on the same plant, the leaves will vary. They are susceptible to the vagaries of time, rainfall, sun and weather. The same is true of our bodies. How revelatory, then, that our bodies need individualized care, particularly when they falter after exposure to the factory-model of medicine.

Please understand that I deeply value some of the gifts offered by conventional medicine. This system of medicine was developed to address crises. If I had a major accident and required surgery, I definitely would want the very best that conventional medicine has to offer. The conventional medical world is the height of the "sick" model of medicine: If the body is ailing, cut, remove, burn, modulate or otherwise alter the current vector the body is traveling.

"*Allo-*," as in *allo*pathic medicine, means "opposite" or "contrary." If the body is traveling in a direction other than we want, then we choose a different direction. We reach for *anti*-biotics, *anti*-inflammatories, *anti*-hypertensives; we aim in the opposite direction of where our body seems to want to go.

Sadly, much of the need for the "*anti-*" therapies results from our own abuse of the body. Heart disease, one of the major killers in industrial countries, is, for the most part, a self-generated condition. The heart falters after years of poor nourishment, little exercise and chemical exposures. After disabling the body through our own activities, we look to the conventional medical world to save us from ourselves. We welcome the "*anti-*" drugs as a panacea to reverse our destructive behavior.

In contrast, Classical Medicine is aimed at augmenting the body's innate vitality. Classical Medicine still harbors the wisdom of how to rebuild the body after major trauma or damage, or to reverse the accumulated effects of poor health care choices. Conventional Medicine has, for the most part, lost this wisdom. Some conventional physicians stumble across the more ancient principles, often out of desperation, and hold their prizes high as if they have discovered a new mother lode. In truth, that wisdom has been there all along, patiently waiting for us to rediscover the treasure chest of healing knowledge available to us since antiquity.

These cures are not flashy; they don't command high-dollar price tags. They are simple and "lowly" and, therefore, often overlooked.

I have a patient in her late sixties who has smoked cigarettes and guzzled coffee since she was a young teenager. Now she is struggling with cardio-obstructive pulmonary disease (COPD) and severe anxiety. When I suggested that this petite, 90-pound woman reduce her daily intake of 12 cups of coffee (!), she shook her head. "The doctor says this anxiety doesn't have anything to do with what I eat or drink," she declared.

I was stunned. In the industrial medical system that rules at this time, the general thinking is that what we take into our bodies has nothing to do with how the body functions. This same post-Industrial Revolution society, however, understands that treating a plastic, metal and rubber machine poorly will hasten *its* demise. In the computer world we say, "Garbage in, garbage out." Why do we consider our own bodies, infinitely more intricate, to be immune from the same laws that govern machines?

What we put into our bodies has everything to do with our health and so does the way we interact with ourselves (thoughts and feelings), our neighbors (communication) and our world (faith and ideology).

Our bodies are not mechanized islands, immune to interaction with the world around us. They represent a reflection of our choices and our genetics. We can influence even the seemingly immutable world of inherited genetic information.

Choosing Green Medicine roots us in a rich, profoundly wise and diverse array of healing substances and practices. The conventional medical world increases our dependence on petroleum (the synthetic base of most pharmaceutical medicines), big business and top-heavy government.

Although conventional medicine was built to address sickness, not health, it offers the current peak of technological sick care when the body is badly damaged. Take the gifts that medical system has to offer and honor them, but don't expect conventional medicine to do things it was never designed to do, such as restore health—only Green Medicine can do that.

PARADIGM OF HEALTH AND DISEASE

Outlined below is a profound paradigm developed by Dr. Jared Zeff that explains the development of disease. The model also suggests how to reverse the disease process and return to a state of health.

Deeply understanding and applying this structure will help you to unify a wide range of medicines and therapies. I think of this structure as a sturdy tie that unites an otherwise unruly pile of sticks. Without this unifying bond, the natural remedies you take are like a collection of mismatched socks: They need a unifying structure so that the body can effectively utilize their healing potential.

Keep in mind that a model is not necessarily the "truth." A wise teacher once said that we entertain ourselves with models until the truth reveals itself. Although the following paradigm may not represent absolute truth, I have seen this model accurately reflect the progression of disease and the restoration of health over and over again.

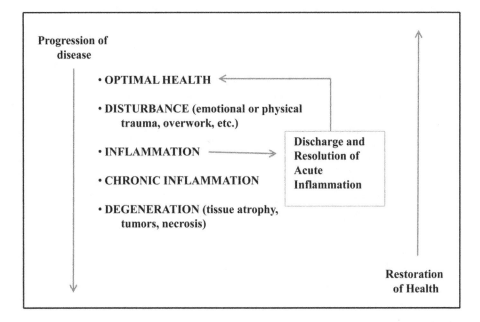

I have observed the accuracy of this model for nearly two decades of clinical practice. The outline provides a simple, elegant understanding of health, illness and healing that is a major source of guidance for me in my work with my own and patients' health.

Most of us begin life in a state of optimal health. Through the course of living, we are exposed to conditions that disturb our equilibrium and challenge the body beyond its ability to compensate. The body responds by generating inflammation (rubor, dolor, calor and tumor—redness, pain, heat and swelling). Fever is one of the most common inflammatory responses.

Inflammation is the body's way of discharging a disturbance from the body. If the body is allowed to complete the inflammatory response, the disturbance is discharged and the body returns to optimal health:

Optimal Health → Disturbance → Inflammation → Discharge →
Optimal Health

Natural therapeutics, when properly applied, speed up the discharge phase and hasten the return to health. Unfortunately, most people attempt to stop the inflammatory response before it has a chance to discharge the disturbance from the body. Stopping or suppressing the inflammation can drive the disturbance deeper into the body, causing chronic irritation. If chronic irritation continues long enough, the body tissues begin to degenerate (resulting in atrophy, tumors and necrosis).

> Optimal Health → Disturbance → Inflammation → Suppression → Chronic Inflammation → Tissue Degeneration

A classic example of suppression of inflammation, recognized by conventional as well as Classical Medicine, is applying cortisone cream to eczema rashes. Cortisone stops inflammation by suppressing the activity of the immune system. Patients with eczema who apply cortisone creams often develop asthma (or asthma worsens, if they already have the condition) as the eczema improves. In essence, the cortisone cream suppresses the eczema and drives the inflammation deeper into the body—in this case, to the lungs.

Patients often notice that, as their asthma improves, the eczema returns—the body has strengthened to the point of pushing the inflammation to the surface (skin) once again (see the "Laws of Cure" in Chapter 2). They reapply the cortisone cream; the eczema improves; and the asthma worsens. This chronic cycle of suppression and improvement may continue for years before the body becomes too weary to push the inflammation back to the surface any longer. At that point, the eczema diminishes to a low-grade irritation, as the asthma becomes a more deep-seated, chronic condition.

Natural therapeutics, when improperly applied, can also cause suppression of inflammation and irritation. Although suppression is less likely with natural therapeutics, a practitioner of hydrotherapy, herbs and/or homeopathic remedies must be mindful and watch carefully for any signs of suppression. In the example given above, asthma is a "chronic irritation" of the lung tissue caused by suppressing a surface irritation. In Classical Medicine, the surface irritation (eczema) is a less serious condition than chronic inflammation in a vital organ (asthma). If the chronic inflammation continues long enough, lung tissues will degenerate.

Generally, the body will not develop measurable signs of damage until the disease has reached the "chronic inflammation" or "degeneration" level. Taking a biopsy of an acutely infected sinus, for example, and examining the tissue under a microscope usually will not reveal major tissue changes. A chronically infected sinus, however, will show signs of irritation at the cellular level. Long-term irritation may cause degeneration of the tissues. Necrosis is a late-stage manifestation of tissue degeneration.

The model for returning to health is a reversal of the disease process.

Degeneration → Chronic Inflammation → Inflammation → Discharge → Optimal Health

Different classical medical systems focus on diverse methods to stimulate this reversal. Chiropractic medicine, for example, focuses on normal spinal alignment as a central key to restoring health. When the spine is well-aligned, all of the nerve roots exiting the spine can properly enervate internal organs, thereby optimizing their function. Chinese and Ayurvedic medicine aim to balance different elements within the body, utilizing a variety of treatments including diet, herbs, massage and acupuncture.

Naturopathic medicine aims to restore the digestive tract first, by two central methods—proper nutrition and hydrotherapy. The digestive system is responsible for absorption of nutrients and disposal of most wastes in the body. If the digestive system is functioning optimally, the body has a fighting chance of receiving all the nutrition available in the food we eat and disposing of all the wastes generated by the body during the natural processes of maintenance and repair.

Constitutional hydrotherapy—a specific hydrotherapy treatment designed to stimulate the immune system and increase circulation in the digestive system—is the simplest, most powerful and least expensive method of healing the digestive tract. (See "Hydrotherapy" section of Chapter 2.)

Dietary changes and constitutional hydrotherapy treatments also stimulate something our current medical terminology has no tools to measure: the body's innate healing ability. As the body strengthens, the disease process begins to reverse itself. Degeneration improves to the level of chronic irritation and then chronic irritation becomes acute—the body finally has enough energy to "clean house," or to bring the acute inflammation that was suppressed back to the surface. Often the acute inflammation returns in the form of a low-grade fever, or a cold or flu-like illness, that lasts for a couple of days. Sometimes the housecleaning, also referred to as the "healing crisis," manifests as the return of an old illness. In contrast to earlier episodes, however, the healing crisis usually is much briefer and less intense than the original occurrence.

If allowed to run its course, the acute inflammation allows the body to discharge the original disturbance and it returns once again to a state of optimal health. When the body finally mounts an acute inflammation after a long, chronic illness, remember that the inflammation must be allowed to run its course without any further suppression (e.g., no cortisone or aspirin).

In addition to nutrition and hydrotherapy, many other treatments stimulate the body's innate healing ability. Homeopathy, botanical medicines, stress reduction, acupuncture and physical therapies all may support the body in its healing journey. Inner work, meditation and counseling address the roots of some illnesses. Choosing a particular modality requires both skill and intuition—a practitioner needs a solid knowledge of his or her subject and a well-honed intuition to select the method or methods that will most benefit a patient. Often I tell patients that we will be doing some "detective work" to discover what treatments will be most catalytic for them. Of course, the response depends, in part, on the skill of the practitioner and on his or her ability to utilize a particular healing tool.

This marriage of knowledge and intuition is paramount for application of these principles at home. Learn everything you can about the modalities you find most useful, or to which you feel most drawn. Consult local practitioners; read and study. Practice what you are learning. Information becomes living knowledge when you apply the information in your life. Learn to listen to your intuition, the "natural intelligence" that guides the application of knowledge. Remember that each person is different; what affects one person may not affect another. As you become more familiar with your own and your family's bodies, you will make better and better selections based on your healing knowledge.

CHAPTER 2

Greening Your Medicine Chest

I am offering you a treasure chest filled to the brim with jewels that are inexpensive, effective and easy to use. By investing a few minutes a day, you can quickly build physical, mental, emotional and spiritual health to a degree that may have eluded you in the past.

My aim is to share as much as I can in these pages to shorten your learning curve so that you can create health for yourself and your loved ones. I want to ignite your appreciation and respect for the variety of natural medicinal therapies available for constructing and renovating your health.

DEEP LISTENING

The ability to listen deeply to the body and its needs will guide you in selecting which treatment or supplement to use. Rarely does a single factor cause disease; usually, many events and circumstances have contributed to an illness. Similarly, many tools may be needed to restore optimal health.

Your ability to listen deeply to your body will guide you to the most appropriate tool(s) for your situation. I might have 10 patients with a cold, for example and send them home with 10 different treatment protocols. I am making treatment recommendations for *the person* who has the cold, as well as for the illness itself.

Deep listening will guide you in choosing the correct remedies for your body, according to its needs *at that time*. The cold you developed in September might require completely different therapies than a cold the following spring. Approach each condition and each situation with fresh eyes.

EMBRACING THE FULL SPECTRUM OF HEALING THERAPIES

Think of medicine as a spectrum ranging from charcoal to diamond. Both charcoal and diamond are composed of nothing but carbon. Drugs and surgery populate the charcoal end of the spectrum. Food, herbs and nutritional supplements fall in the middle range. Energetic therapies, such as acupuncture, visualization, color therapy, aromatherapy and homeopathy, populate the "diamond" end of the spectrum.

Each of us has a natural "home base" along this spectrum. Most of the therapies I utilize range from the middle-to-the-diamond end of the spectrum. On occasion, though, I will prescribe pharmaceutical drugs, or encourage a patient to pursue surgery.

Some might consider this heresy. I call it common sense. Someone may come to me *thinking* the diamond end of the spectrum is where he or she belongs; their body, however, may require charcoal therapies. Even people whose "home base" is the diamond end may need to dip into the carbon end of the spectrum from time to time to address a particular condition.

Karen, a dear friend, recently was diagnosed with a very aggressive form of cervical cancer. She had been bleeding heavily for over a year, which is not uncommon during peri-menopause. As soon as I knew about the bleeding, I begged Karen to have more testing (uterine ultrasound, endometrial biopsy, etc.). She refused. As a clairvoyant, she was extremely sensitive to her surroundings. She had undergone several difficult experiences in her lifetime with domineering, all-knowing conventional physicians. Karen wanted nothing to do with them or their testing methods.

We had several long discussions about utilizing conventional medicine where it shines—in this case, testing technology to determine the cause of her bleeding.

"Having the tests done does not mean you are wedded to doing drugs and surgery," I reminded my friend.

Karen smiled patiently and did not reply. I knew she was not willing to endure the contact with conventional doctors to have the tests done.

Finally, after a year of episodic heavy bleeding, Karen hemorrhaged. In the early morning hours, her partner drove her to the hospital. He stayed by her side as the reports began to come in—a tumor in the adnexa region, possibly invading the pelvic area. The gynecologist suspected an aggressive form of cancer, complicated by severe anemia from her long episodes of bleeding.

Karen called me, seeking my advice about whether or not to accept the blood transfusion.

"The horse is out of the barn at this point," I said gently. "The body has gone beyond the point it can restore itself without outside help." I encouraged her to accept the blood transfusion.

That day Karen began a long journey that led, thankfully, to complete eradication of the cancer. Initially, she completely resisted any offerings from the conventional medical world.

"I hate those arrogant doctors!" she blurted out. "I can cure this cancer without their help." Karen was determined she could meditate away the five-centimeter tumor. Although I know people who have succeeded in using energetic therapies (the diamond end of the spectrum) to heal major diseases, I was doubtful that, in her weakened state, the energetic therapies alone would cure the cancer. If she had pursued testing and discovered the tumor at an earlier stage, she might have been successful with energetic therapies alone.

Karen's natural place on the healing spectrum was definitely toward the diamond end. At that point, though, she needed to dip into the charcoal end of the spectrum to address her advanced condition. By combining diamond spectrum therapies with the charcoal treatments, she was better able to tolerate the side effects of conventional therapies. She made the best use of several therapies along the spectrum.

EMBRACE DIVERSITY IN YOUR TREATMENT CHOICES

I have worked with fundamentalists at both ends of the spectrum. Most conventional physicians truly believe that "charcoal" medicines are the only valid medical treatments. I also know practitioners at the diamond end of the spectrum who have a vendetta against "charcoal" medicine. These classical practitioners instruct patients to pursue only one particular treatment modality (theirs, of course!) in the pursuit of health. Many classical homeopaths, for example, tell patients to use single homeopathic remedies and absolutely no other therapies, particularly "energetic" therapies, while they are pursuing homeopathic treatment. This rigid, dogmatic approach to homeopathy is an aberration of Dr. Samuel Hahnemann's teachings.

Hahnemann, the modern founder of homeopathy, instructed patients in removing "the obstacles to cure" before taking constitutional homeopathic remedies. Those "obstacles" might include nutritional deficiencies, lack of exercise, dehydration, poor digestion, food reactions and/or environmental exposures. Hahnemann offered counsel on how to eliminate these obstacles before pursuing more subtle forms of treatment.

At times you may discover that a single remedy or one treatment modality absolutely is the optimal choice. Honor that wisdom, too. I'm simply encouraging you to keep your mind and heart open to the many possibilities of restoring balance and, therefore, health.

Marrying a philosophy blinds me to my needs in the moment. I can't see what would be best for me, right here and now, if I'm wedded to certain treatments.

DEVELOP NEW "REFLEXES" FOR HEALTH CARE

We also choose therapies out of habit. Most of us have been trained in the "take this for that" mentality. Take Tylenol for a fever; take Pepto-Bismol for a stomach ache. We don't stop to consider the root of a symptom; we simply want it to go away.

Many of the therapies in this toolbox fall in the middle of the medical spectrum, about half-way between the charcoal and the diamond ends of the spectrum. Some, such as deep breathing, meditation, homeopathy and flower essences, populate the diamond end of the spectrum. Learn these treatments and make them a part of your daily life. You will be learning a way of working with your body that supports both you and the Earth.

UNIFYING PRINCIPLES FOR CLASSICAL MEDICINES

Although each system of Classical Medicine has developed different treatment modalities, they all share the same philosophy. The following principles describe classical modalities as diverse as chiropractic treatment and meditation, acupuncture and intravenous chelation therapy.

Vis Medicatrix Naturae: The healing power of nature

All living things have the ability to grow, regenerate and repair. In contrast, a dented chair will not repair itself. My own body has a living blueprint that guides the restoration process. Classical medical therapies aim to engage and augment this healing ability, rather than trying to override the body's efforts in righting itself.

When engaged, this innate healing ability can be fostered and accelerated. Instead of over-riding this wisdom, Classical Medicine aims to enhance the body's efforts to repair itself.

Tolle Causum: Identify and treat the cause

Rather than cover symptoms, Classical Medicine searches for the root of the condition. Chinese medicine, for example, addresses the root (*ben*) as well as the branches (*biao*) of a disease. The branches are the immediate symptoms. Yes, we do want immediate relief from discomfort. Treating only the leaves, however, would leave the diseased roots to fester. Once the body responds to palliative care (the leaves), we expand the focus to include the roots of the disease.

One patient came to me seeking treatment for chronic bronchitis. He was mystified about why he was having repeated respiratory infections. He was a professional athlete who had always been in good health.

I asked about any changes in his life—anything that might have contributed to this sudden transformation. I was not surprised to learn that, in the past nine months, his life had undergone several volcanic changes.

"Last June my wife went into the hospital with an undiagnosed viral illness," Stephen recounted. "She was five months pregnant. The doctors weren't very worried. 'A couple of days of bed rest and she'll be fine,' they told me. We consulted a psychic who said the same thing.

"Well, three days later, both she and the baby died. I was left alone with my six-year-old daughter.

"I sold my house and bought an RV. My daughter and I lived with my parents for a couple of months and then I moved out here. I'm in a new relationship now, with a woman who has four kids. We're engaged, and my daughter and I are in the process of packing to move into her house."

I drew in a deep breath. "Wow, Stephen, no wonder your body is reeling."

"What do you mean?" he asked, looking perplexed. "I'm strong. I'm used to dealing with tough situations; I'm an athlete. It's not that big a deal."

When I checked his pulses and tongue, aspects of Chinese diagnosis, I noted his tongue was a bright purple color. Purple indicates stagnation, which leads to pain, whether physical or emotional. I knew from the color of this patient's tongue that he was still in pain—still grieving the loss of his wife and unborn child. Although his mind had moved on, his body and soul were still struggling.

Over the next month we addressed his physical as well as emotional symptoms. His lungs, the seat of grief in Chinese medicine, began to improve. We talked about his future plans and the possibility of reconsidering the pace of the changes he was making. His tongue gradually changed from bright to lighter purple. At the end of the month, the tongue wasn't back to a normal pink color, but it was much improved.

Our minds often override the deeper messages from our bodies and spirits. If I had simply administered acupuncture, herbs and supplements, I would have missed the root of this patient's illness. Addressing only the branches—in this case, the chronic bronchitis—probably would not have resolved the symptoms completely. He needed to come to grips with the magnitude of life changes he was undergoing, as well as finish grieving the loss of his wife and unborn child before his lungs could completely recover.

First do no harm

One of the great blessings of many "green" medicines is that, usually, at their very worst, *they will do nothing harmful.* The conventional medical world utilizes powerful drugs in their "arsenal"—yes, that's the word commonly used to describe treatments. Admittedly, this language of weaponry is used by other medical systems as well. Most of the conventional medical treatments are not catalysts; they are cannons. Some conditions truly require cannons, like Karen whose cervical dysplasia had progressed to carcinoma. Many ailments, however, require nourishment, not guns. Imagine firing a canon at a hangnail—not a very appropriate use of force.

My aim is always to gently catalyze the body before slamming it. Again and again, I am amazed at how simple, elegant treatments can effect great change in the body.

I have an elderly patient, a very active 79-year-old, who has had gastric problems for many years. She has tried a host of supplements and herbs, without great success. We decided to test her for constitutional food intolerances, a simple test that looks for the *primary* food or food group that causes inflammation in the gut. To her surprise, eggs tested as her primary intolerance. Within a week of eliminating eggs, her gastric pain resolved and her loose stools returned to normal.

The next step is to rebuild the digestive tract, using the constitutional hydrotherapy treatment (see page 55) to strengthen the digestive tract so that she is no longer reactive to eggs, or any other foods. Then we will be addressing the deepest root of her gastric issues.

If I were not willing or able to do the detective work to discover the root of this patient's digestive problems, she likely would have been happy to continue taking fistfuls of supplements. I'm not satisfied, however, with stopping there, because supplements can be used to "Band-Aid" symptoms just as pharmaceutical drugs can. While the supplements have fewer side effects they can, when well-prescribed, help to rebuild the body. Stopping at supplements alone, though, would have missed the root of the condition.

Doctor as Teacher

The Latin word for doctor is *docere*, meaning "to teach." The primary role of a doctor is to educate patients, to give them information to improve their own health.

This desire to teach patients to achieve greater levels of health has spurred me to create books, CDs, DVDs and other teaching materials, to support patients in fulfilling their own vision of health.

This view of doctor as teacher also inspires me to create a collaborative relationship with patients. I am not the doctor-god, dictating behavior and prescribing medicines for a patient. Instead, I work with a patient to fulfill his or her vision of health. This is a radically different approach from what most of us grew up with.

Prevention

I laugh when my "sick" care insurance agent tells me the company will pay for an annual "wellness" visit. In truth, the visit is not aimed at preventing disease, but rather diagnosing illness at an earlier stage. The company hopes that early discovery will minimize the cost of treatment. While this approach does not improve my health, it does detect the initial warning signs of disease.

Prevention requires studying health even more closely than the processes of disease. True preventive medicine involves making daily investments in our health—eating foods that nourish our bodies, exercising, developing loving relationships and supportive communities and contributing to the health of the Earth. Healthy people live in healthy environments. Preventive medicine means working for clean air, land and water; human health is inseparable from the health of the planet.

Treat the Whole Person

When Betty walked into my office, her eyes were red and puffy and her shoulders hunched forward. Usually, Betty gave me a bear hug; that day she quietly took a seat across from me.

"I'm here for high blood pressure," she explained.

After gathering some information, I touched Betty's arm. "What's going on in your life?" I asked. "Why do you think you are ill right now?"

Betty burst into tears. She and her husband were considering retirement, which involved selling the dairy farm that had been the center of their lives for the last 40 years. "It just tears me up to think about leaving that place," said Betty, "and I'm not sure how I'm going to get along with my husband when we move into a smaller place."

She shook her head. "You know, when I saw my insurance plan provider about the high blood pressure, she lectured me about taking hormone replacement therapy. She never asked about what was going on in my life. She just wanted to get me on estrogen therapy."

That day Betty's treatment involved stress-reduction techniques, herbs and dietary changes. Cleary, the herbs alone would not have corrected her high blood pressure.

As illuminated in the paradigm of health and disease, the healing process may cause unresolved wounds from the past to resurface. Such wounding may have occurred on physical, mental, emotional and/or spiritual levels. Focusing on healing any aspect of the self can activate past disease. As the body strengthens, it accrues enough energy to "clean house"—to bring forth, examine and discharge past garbage.

Each individual follows a unique path in restoring health and wholeness. Although individual, certain patterns typify that path. The template of healing outlined below is common to all forms of Classical Medicine.

THE LAWS OF CURE

Healing occurs

- from inside to outside (internal organs first, skin last)
- from top to bottom (from the head to the feet)
- from most recent to most distant (recent symptoms recur first, followed by older symptoms—in other words, in reverse chronological order)
- from least important to most important organs

THE GREEN MEDICINE CHEST: CLASSICAL THERAPIES FOR YOUR MEDICINE CHEST

- Food
- Herbs
- Homeopathic Remedies

- Essential Oils
- Flower Essences
- Hydrotherapy
- Castor Oil Packs
- Skin Brushing
- Acupressure
- Breathing Exercises
- Qigong
- Meditation and Guided Relaxation
- Indigenous Medicine

FOOD

The doctor of the future will give no medicine, but will instruct his patient in the care of the human frame, in diet and in the cause and prevention of disease.

HENRY FORD
"Wizard Edison", *The Newark Advocate*
(2 January 1903), p. 1.

Food is your best medicine. All of the fancy pills, supplements, herbs and other potions will never compensate for a lack of vital, nutritious food.

Your food choices must be individualized for your particular body. Healthy food for *you* may be poison for someone else. I learned the importance of individualizing my food choices at a fairly young age. Many of the wonderful, "healthy" foods that I was eating were *not* healthy for my particular body.

Ideally, you would consult with a health care provider who can work with you to create an individualized diet to address your particular health needs. In the Appendices, you will find contact information if you are interested in pursuing specific testing (constitutional food intolerance, IgG allergy and ALCAT testing) to assess which foods nourish your particular body.

The following guidelines will assist you in choosing foods that support health.

- **Choose foods that are as close as possible to their natural state**. Apples, for example, are harvested directly from trees; apple turnovers are not.

- **Choose organic foods**. Recent research demonstrates that organic foods contain about 70 percent more nutrients than their convention- ally grown counterparts. Some organic foods cost more. This is, in part, because many of the hidden costs—e.g., replenishing the soil and avoiding soil erosion through appropriate watering techniques—are accounted for by organic food growers. In addition, most government subsidies go to agribusiness giants instead of smaller, more efficient organic farms. Choosing organic foods supports the health of the land and all its inhabitants, as well as our own bodies.

- **Eat local foods**. Buying and eating local foods again supports our own bodies as well as the health of the land. Eating locally means that we are ingesting food grown from the soil where we live. We literally become calibrated to the land, containing a similar ratio of minerals and nutrients to the soil we live upon and with. We also reduce fossil fuel consumption by eating local foods. Instead of buying Granny Smith apples grown in New Zealand, flown thousands of miles and then trucked even farther to our local supermarket, we're buying food that has traveled less than 10 miles.

- Barbara Kingsolver, author of *Animal, Vegetable, Miracle* (Harper-Collins, 2007), notes that "each food item in a typical U.S. meal has traveled an average of 1500 miles. . . . If every U.S. citizen ate just one meal a week (any meal) composed of locally and organically raised meats and produce, we would reduce our country's oil consumption by over 1.1 million barrels of oil *every week*. That's not gallons, but barrels. Small changes in buying habits can make big differences. Becoming a less energy-dependent nation may just need to start with a good breakfast."

- **Choose seasonal foods**. In Chinese medicine, they (gently) divide the world according to five elements. A more accurate way to describe these elements would be to say these five "phases" weave the fabric of the world. Each element is associated with a season, a color, an organ, a planet, an animal, etc. This complex system, so elegantly related, offers profound wisdom on eating seasonal foods: the foods that come in season at certain times of the year support the organs the body focuses on during that season.

  In the spring, the body "leans" more on the liver and gallbladder. The plants that begin to push from the muddy earth at that time of year are wonderful supports for the liver. Dandelion greens, plantain leaves, arugula and other bitter greens stimulate bile secretion, helping to clear the effects of a winter spent eating heavier, greasier foods.

During the summer, the body emphasizes heart function. This fiery organ is cooled by the more watery fruits and vegetables that come in season during the summer: zucchini, lettuce, green beans and Swiss chard.

As summer passes into Indian summer (the fifth season, not officially recognized in the West), winter squash and grains begin to ripen. These denser, more nutrient-rich foods support the stomach and spleen, the digestive organs the body focuses on during this season of golden light and cool nights.

In the autumn, the body "leans" more on the lungs and large intestine. Not surprisingly, this is the season when colds and the flu become more common. Aromatic herbs and foods support lung and large intestine health during this season of cool, damp weather.

In the winter, when food is less abundant on land, we traditionally relied on food from the sea—seaweed or sea vegetables and fish. These saltwater foods support the kidneys and bladder, the organs the body emphasizes more in the winter.

Or course, all of these organs are working all year round. During certain seasons, though, the body emphasizes certain ones. Giving the "seasonal" organ more support during that time will help support overall health throughout the year.

- Avoid Genetically Modified Organisms (GMO), or what I call "Frankenfoods." Many corn and canola crops now are grown from GMO seeds developed by Monsanto. Some GMO crops were developed to "grow" insulin and other pharmaceutical medicines. Others contain genes that make the plant resistant to Round-Up, a toxic herbicide used to kill weeds. Normal corn or canola crops sprayed with Round-Up die; the GMO crops survive. Unfortunately, seed from these GMO plants is spreading to surrounding fields and contaminating other corn and canola crops. The U.S. Food and Drug Administration (FDA) has ignored many studies that demonstrate that humans develop bizarre symptoms and many animals die when exposed to GMO crops.

- Choose foods low on the food chain. Animals concentrate chemicals in their fat and lymphatic tissue, which explains why birds of prey have much higher levels of DDT, PCBs and other toxic chemicals than seed-eating birds. Eat grains, legumes and vegetables more frequently than fish or meat.

- Consider the following general guidelines in choosing the types of food you eat. Remember that this information needs to be individualized, to meet your particular nutritional needs.

  - 60 percent grains and legumes
  - 30 percent fruits and vegetables
  - 10 percent meat, cheese, eggs, tofu and other concentrated protein sources

- Most Americans eat far too much animal protein. The more animal protein you eat, the more uric acid you produce. Breaking down and excreting uric acid weakens the kidneys over time. Eating more animal protein acidifies the body, increases calcium loss and generally inflames the body.

- All food sources, including plant foods, contain protein. The World Health Organization recommends eating 50 grams of protein per day, with increased amounts for pregnant or lactating women.

- 10-to-15 percent of your daily calorie intake should come from fats. The average Westerner consumes about 40 percent of his or her calories as fat!

- The type of fat or oil you eat is as important as the quantity. Eliminate altered fats (rancid or hydrogenated fats and oils) from your diet. These include margarines and shortenings, whether they are used fresh, or included in processed and deep-fried foods. Keep saturated animal fats to a minimum. Include cold-pressed oils in your diet. Keep all oils, including olive oil, in the refrigerator: heat, light and air cause oils to become rancid.

- Read labels. Information is power, and this simple step can radically change your food choices and, therefore, your health. "Evaporated cane juice," for example, is the new euphemism for sugar—doesn't that sound so much healthier? No matter what the name, as little as a gram of sugar will depress immune function up to 24 hours. Be a smart shopper; read the label and choose foods that are nutrient-rich, without additives, preservatives or simple sugars. A general rule of thumb: If you have trouble pronouncing the name of an ingredient, you probably don't want to ingest it. Propylene glycol, for example, makes ice cream and other products feel "creamy" in your mouth. This chemical is also used to de-ice airplanes.

- Take time to chew. Chew every bite of food as many as 50 times. This first step in the digestive process grinds food into smaller pieces and mixes saliva with the food. Saliva contains amylase, an enzyme that begins carbohydrate digestion. Simply chewing food can resolve a host of digestive complaints.

Early in my years of practice, I worked with a patient with late-stage pancreatic cancer. My primary focus with this very motivated patient was to use acupuncture for pain control. His physical therapist was teaching him qigong, and he listened to guided visualization tapes each evening.

One day he asked me for dietary recommendations. We discussed the importance of eating vital, nutrient-rich foods to support the body. I suggested he eliminate cane and beet sugar that directly feed cancer cells. I also encouraged him to eliminate food coloring and additives, many of which are known carcinogens.

When I arrived a week later, he was eating a Snickers bar as his wife heated up Campbell's mushroom soup. I looked puzzled as he happily chewed on the candy bar.

"I talked to my oncologist about diet," he explained. "The oncologist says it doesn't matter what I eat; that has no effect on my body or the disease."

I was too stunned to speak. What I wanted to say was, "Sure, what you eat doesn't matter *if you're planning to die.*" I knew this patient was already far progressed in the disease. To be charitable to the oncologist, I'm assuming he wanted the patient to be as comfortable as possible in his final days. Why should the patient worry about his food choices when he was facing death? On a more realistic note, the oncologist probably never had any nutritional training in medical school.

Sadly, this patient continued eating canned soup and chocolate bars and died a few weeks later. Certainly, diet was not the only factor that contributed to his passing. His lack of nourishing foods, though, made his final days less comfortable and may even have hastened his death.

Food also has a profound effect on our mental and emotional well-being. *Psychodietetics* (Stein & Day Publishers, 1974), was one of the first books to popularize scientific research about how food affects our thinking processes and our emotions. Numerous studies since that time have demonstrated how food affects behavior and mood, particularly in children.

Food intolerances versus food allergies

Food allergies: True food allergies are caused by immune globulin E (IgE) or immune globulin G (IgG) reactions in the body. If you are allergic to oranges, for example, the body produces immune globulin E or immune globulin G to "attack" the orange food particles. Many other tissues are caught in the crossfire, causing a wide range of symptoms (see below). IgE reactions are immediate, hypersensitivity reactions, e.g., throat and bronchial swelling, hives and difficulty breathing. These "anaphylactic" symptoms usually occur within seconds or minutes of ingesting a food. In contrast, IgG reactions are delayed hypersensitivity reactions and may occur four hours to four *days* after ingesting a food.

Most people already are aware of the immediate, IgE food reactions. The delayed IgG reactions are more difficult to detect. Who would think that the headache on Thursday might be related to the tomato soup one ate on Monday?

Food intolerances cause inflammatory reactions in the body, but they are not necessarily mediated by the immune system. Food intolerances can be assessed in many ways:

ALCAT (antigen leukocyte cellular antibody testing): tests the final common inflammatory pathway in the body; i.e., it looks for *any* type of inflammatory response. This test looks for any and all food reactions and rates them as severe, moderate, mild, or no reaction.

Constitutional food intolerance testing: assesses the *primary* food or food group that inflames the digestive tract, particularly the liver. The test also looks for any food combinations that cause an inflammatory response.

EAV and other electrical testing devices: Many different types of machines measure the electrical "current" or electromagnetic field in the body, usually utilizing particular acupuncture points. If the current is diminished when a particular food or substance is introduced, it is considered detrimental. If the current remains the same or increases, the substance is considered supportive.

Muscle testing: Also known as "applied kinesiology," this form of testing utilizes a patient's muscle strength to determine whether a food is supportive or detrimental for the body. If the muscle remains "strong" while a patient is holding a food, then the food is supportive for the body. If the muscle goes "weak," then the food is considered detrimental. This testing method requires great skill on the practitioner's part, because the results are very easily influenced. Because the results are so easily biased, I do not recommend this form of food testing.

Common food intolerance and allergy reactions

Anxiety	Fatigue
Arthritis	Hay Fever symptoms (year-round)
Asthma	Headaches (tension type and migraine)
Attention Deficit Hyperactivity Disorder (ADHD)	Infertility
Autism	Inflammatory Bowel Disease
Bed-wetting	Migraine
Chronic diarrhea	Muscle aches
Chronic Fatigue	Obesity
Depression	Panic attacks
Diabetes	Stuffy nose
Ear or other frequent infections	Urticaria (skin itching, hives)
Eczema	Weight gain

Food is the foundation of your health. Celebrate it as a source of nourishment, joy and pleasure. The more you are able to support your health with your diet, the less you will need to rely on other supplements or treatments to bolster your body, mind and spirit.

HERBS

In ancient times, humans learned what foods to eat and what medicines to prepare by watching animals, particularly the bear. Of all the North American and European animals, the bear most closely resembles humans. Many plant names honor this relationship with bear, e.g., bearberry, or *Uva ursi*. *Ursi* is Latin for "bear."

The Chippewa, or "Anishnabe" as they call themselves, recognize Bear as a profound teacher of healing wisdom. Long ago Bear came to an Anishnabe village and transformed himself into a human. This elderly man knocked on one of the villagers' door.

"Please help me," the feeble man pleaded. "I am sick."

The woman took in this elderly man and began to care for him. The man instructed her in what food to prepare and what herbs to gather. As soon as he recovered from one disease, he developed another. He, again, patiently guided the woman in how to care for him. He continued this pattern—developing a disease, teaching the woman how to cure it, and then recovering—until he had progressed through every disease known to humanity.

With the training completed, the old man left the village and returned to his bear form.

To this day, among the Northeastern woodland tribes, the Anishnabe are recognized for their deep healing knowledge.

"House calls": Plants as healing allies in your own backyard

Many of us in the West did not grow up with an intact lineage of healing knowledge. AmyLee, a beloved mentor who is a woodland medicine woman, shared her dismay about watching a documentary on the desperately poor families in Appalachia.

"The people were talking about how they were starving, and there they were, sitting on their porches, literally surrounded by food and medicine! There were plants all around them. I gifted the state of West Virginia with a grant proposal to help retrain these people in plant wisdom. I say 're-train,' because many of these people had a family tradition of working with plants for food and medicine. In the last couple of generations, they've lost a lot of that knowledge.

"I have the same reaction when I see a news report about some disaster in a foreign country like Haiti and how the people have no food. And there they are, surrounded by plants! The food and medicine are right there!"

Years ago I interviewed a man who had spent most of his adult life trying to save Enola Hill, a sacred site on the western slopes of Mount Hood in Oregon. This sacred site has been shared by numerous local tribes for millennia. Although not native himself, this man had a deep reverence for the land and the native inhabitants of that area.

"The elders teach," he explained as we walked the sacred sites, still blessed with the marks of the native people who had visited these sites for millennia, "that for every disease known to humanity, there is a cure. Right here, right around us. Every disease has a plant ally that will cure that disease. Native people from this entire region come to this site to gather and prepare herbs for medicine. Of course, some of those plants grow in their local area, and they gather the plants there, too. But this particular area, this wilderness site, has an incredible abundance of healing plants."

Native elders around the world offer the same wisdom: We are surrounded by plant allies that are the ultimate source of our food and medicine. Gathering medicine from our neighborhood supports the health of the land and attunes us with the environment where we live.

I strive as much as possible to treat with herbs from the land where I live, especially the native plants. I do make exceptions, because the Chinese have developed such a profound, synergistic way of preparing herbs. In general, though, I aim for local sources.

Healing Wisdom: Deepening Your Knowledge of Herbs

As recently as a century ago, many people had the good fortune of living in communities where grandmothers, uncles, medicine people and *curanderas* (folk healers) worked with the ancient wisdom of plants. You may be in the process of rediscovering this deeply rooted knowledge. I offer you the following insights to encourage you in that process of discovery. You are embarking on a journey that could last a lifetime. These four steps are common guideposts I have witnessed in my own and others' learning process.

1. "Use this for that." Many people accustomed to seeking conventional medical help are trained to think in terms of one medicine to treat one ailment. Prilosec treats stomach acid, for example, and Prozac treats depression. Take this to treat that. Those beginning to experiment with herbs, homeopathics and nutritional supplements usually bring this same mentality to using natural medicines; e.g., take comfrey to heal bones; use St. Johns Wort for depression.

Few beginners understand that effectively choosing a homeopathic or a botanical medicine requires a completely different paradigm. "Natural," or what I prefer to call "Classical" Medicine, views the *person* who is suffering with a particular condition, rather than a *disease* affecting a particular body. Conventional medicine simply looks at the disease and prescribes this drug to treat that disease. Classical Medicine treats the person who is suffering with a disease. Ten different people with the same medical diagnosis, for example, might take 10 different homeopathic remedies or 10 different combinations of herbs to address their particular set of symptoms.

A common misunderstanding in this first stage of exploration is that only pharmaceutical drugs qualify as "medicine."

One day, while waiting in line at the post office, I happened to meet a patient who had come to me for help with menopausal symptoms several months before. "Oh, that's all taken care of," she explained. "I went to my medical doctor for some medicine." As I left the post office, I wondered what she thought the hormones and herbs I had prescribed were. If they were not "medicine," were they "candy" or "placebos?" Perhaps I had failed to explain that these substances were indeed potent medicines, albeit ones that might take some time to address the hormonal changes she was experiencing.

Many people are accustomed to the lightning-quick action of pharmaceutical drugs. The primary aim of these drugs, however, is to *over-ride*, not support, the body's innate healing processes. Patients may not understand that some natural substances require time to rebalance the body. Of course, some natural medicines can act very quickly, as anyone who has used homeopathic arnica for a badly bruised knee or twisted ankle can verify.

Many natural health care practitioners also rely on the "this for that" model when prescribing natural medicines.

One of my former office partners worked for several years as a pharmaceutical company representative before entering chiropractic school. In her practice, she prescribed many supplements using the same pharmaceutical paradigm. She simply substituted supplements for drugs. "Here, take this for sleep. Take that for sore muscles. Take this for indigestion." She did not understand the importance of balancing nutrients (e.g., always combining calcium with magnesium, or prescribing all of the B-vitamins together rather than in isolation) or tailoring prescriptions for individual patients.

Why, for example, was the patient having trouble sleeping? Was depression an underlying issue? Did the patient eat well, including plenty of B-vitamin-rich whole grains? Did she exercise? Did muscle spasms keep her awake? These concerns were never considered. Most of her patients improved some with her prescriptions, but they did not experience the full potential benefit of the herbs or supplements.

2. Functions and actions of herbs. In this second stage, a student of natural medicine begins to delve into the way a particular herb or nutrient works in the body. Comfrey promotes tissue healing, for example, because it contains a substance called allantoin that stimulates cell division. Plants are conglomerates of many elements with numerous different actions.

"Standardized" preparations of herbs focus on one specific substance in a plant, assuming that one particular element governs the effect of that plant. In truth, though, this is another shading of the "this for that" mentality. No one substance "rules" the action of a plant. Many elements contribute to the way a plant influences our bodies. This complexity explains why a single plant might be prescribed for many different reasons.

Today St. Johns Wort is most commonly prescribed for depression. Twenty years ago, though, it was mainly used for nerve damage and nerve-like pain. St. Johns Wort oil, applied externally, treats burns, sciatic pain and crush injuries (again, related to its effect on the nervous system).

The functions and actions of an herb are discovered through scientific research. Most cutting-edge herbal research is conducted in Germany, where they still have a centuries-old unbroken tradition of using plants as medicine.

3. Energetics of herbs. Discovering the energetic properties of herbs requires stepping outside the Western scientific paradigm and relying on ways of knowing not easily recorded by machines. Chinese herbalists, in particular, have pioneered this branch of botanical medicine over nearly 6,000 years of continuous practice.

The energetic attributes of herbs include such properties as heating, drying, cooling, tonifying and moistening. In Chinese herbalism, plants are classified according to actions; e.g., herbs that "dry dampness," or "clear toxic heat," or "nourish the blood."

Herbs are also grouped according to the internal organs they affect. Rather than relying on guesswork, this information was gleaned by people who had the ability to "see" subtle energetic changes in the body. When someone ingested a particular herb, the sensitive person would "see" a particular organ or acupuncture channel associated with that organ "light up." We do not have scientific instruments in the West that can duplicate these ways of knowing. From my perspective, lacking such machines does not invalidate the information but, rather, highlights the limitations of our current Western technology.

Western herbalism also has an historical tradition of identifying energetic properties of herbs. In the Middle Ages, herbalists commonly discussed these energetic actions. Some of that information has passed by word-of-mouth and written documents into modern times.

Prescribing herbs according to energetic principles requires evaluating the whole person, not just the disease. In Chinese medicine, a practitioner gathers information by asking questions, checking tongue and pulses and then developing a "syndrome picture" that describes the patient's condition from an energetic perspective that is rooted in a deep understanding of organ functions. The Chinese herbalist does not prescribe herbs for a particular "disease"; instead, he or she chooses herbs to treat the syndrome picture, which is gleaned from examining the whole person.

4. Essence or spiritual properties of herbs. One of my beloved teachers was a Chippewa (Anishnabe) man named Sun Bear. His people recognize three major healing traditions within their nation: those who heal by sharing wisdom, those who heal with their hands, and those who heal with herbs. He considered himself mainly a wisdom-healer, but Sun Bear also had a formidable knowledge of herbs and other healing techniques.

During a break in one of his teachings, a woman approached Sun Bear to ask him about the healing properties of a particular herb. Sun Bear paused for a moment and looked quizzically at the woman. "You're a two-legged, just like me," he said finally. "Why don't you go ask the plant?" Sun Bear was describing an ability that I believe most, if not all, humans possess: the ability to quiet our minds and listen deeply to other elements of creation.

Plants, animals, rocks and water are continuously communicating with each other and with us humans. Most of us, though, are too distracted with the busyness of our lives to quiet our minds enough to truly listen.

I offer you these simple exercises to initiate the process of *deep listening:*

DEEP LISTENING MEDITATION

Choose a plant that draws you, that catches your eye, or interests you because of its healing properties. Seat yourself in front of the plant and allow your eyes to focus softly on it. Take a few deep breaths and imagine your thoughts drifting away like clouds blown on a breezy spring day. As you relax, sense you are breathing the very essence of that plant into your heart. Allow your heart to expand and soften until you sense the essence of that plant rooting right in the center of your being.

From this perspective within the plant, allow yourself to experience life. Notice the flow of water and nutrients within your branches. Sense how the surface cells welcome and transform the sun. Notice the movement of nutrients from the earth upward and from the sun downward. Allow yourself to move through the cycles of a day, a season and a year. If you are a perennial, move through several years, noting your growth and the accumulation of experiences. Give yourself plenty of time to explore life from within this plant ally.

When you are ready, bring your attention back to yourself, this point of life and light within the plant. Allow yourself to expand and grow until this green ally is, once again, a seed, a point of life and light, within your own heart. Notice how the plant feels more alive, more vital within your own being. Observe how your relationship with the plant has changed.

If you enjoy drawing and artwork, you can experiment with a variation of this meditation. Place paper, pencils, pens and any other art supplies you may need in front of you. Sit quietly with a plant or flower, gazing with "soft focus" (slightly blurry vision). Breathe the essence of the plant into your heart. With your eyes still softly focused on the plant or flower, pick up a pencil or paintbrush and begin to move your hand over the paper. Allow the plant's essence to guide your hand. You are aiming to portray the "soul" of the plant, its divine essence, not a literal interpretation of its outer form. Continue relaxing, breathing in the plant's essence, as your hand moves over the paper.

You may choose to repeat these exercises over time. Each experience will draw you deeper and deeper into the spiritual essence of plants. The information you receive may surprise you. One friend who tried the first exercise with dandelion later researched the plant's healing properties in several herbal books. "I was shocked," she reported. "The books only scratched the surface. The plant had so much more to say!"

As you become more familiar with this exercise, you may choose other natural objects to attune with, e.g., a rock or seashell. You can also use this exercise to "listen" to pets and other animals. One woman diagnosed her ailing pet chicken this way. When she moved "inside" the chicken in her meditation, she was able to pinpoint the chicken's illness and describe the problem to the vet. As you become more adept, you can also merge with much larger entities, e.g., landscapes, planets, or even stars.

Most native people understand that the Earth and all of her inhabitants "speak." In order to "hear," however, we need hearts quiet enough to listen to the wordless language. This quiet, respectful approach to listening is part of being in right relationship with self, community and spirit, all of which are vital for full, vibrant health.

For a recorded version of the Deep Listening meditation, please visit *http://www.drjudithboice.com/plantmeditation.html.*

Herbal preparations

You can take herbs in several forms. Each of them is appropriate at different times to accomplish different objectives.

Tea: Prepare tea by placing fresh or dried herbs in a teapot and covering them with boiling water. Let them steep for at least 10 minutes before drinking. This method works best for the leaf or flower of plants and herbs (e.g., peppermint leaves, yarrow blossoms, red clover blossoms, etc.). Teas are a wonderful choice when you need to increase fluid intake, e.g., during a bladder infection or cold.

Decoction: For thicker, woodier parts of the plants, e.g., roots and/or stems, you will need to decoct the tea. Place the roots or twigs in a pot. Cover with fresh water, bring to a boil and then simmer for 10-to-15 minutes. There are a few exceptions to the rule of decocting roots; e.g., marshmallow roots are best left in cold water overnight to extract the medicinal properties of the root.

Poultice: For external application, bruise or crush the leaves or pulverize them in a blender. Place the macerated plant material on a cloth and then apply to the body. These applications are best prepared with fresh herbs. Comfrey leaf and/or root, for example, may be prepared as a poultice to speed the healing of muscle strains and fractures. Be careful about applying poultices on open wounds, however. Some herbs must be applied only after the wound has closed and developed a scab.

Oil: Some herbal remedies are best prepared by "steeping" the plant in oil, usually for several days. One of my favorite oil preparations is *Hypericum perforatum*, or St. John's Wort oil. This plant's common name is derived from the time it blooms, usually on the summer solstice, or "Saint John's Mass" in the Catholic Church. "Wort" means "plant" in Old English; hence, "St. John's Wort" means "Saint John's plant, blooming on the day set aside to honor him."

I love to gather the small, daisy-like yellow blossoms on a sunny summer day, place them in a jar and cover them with olive or other natural vegetable oil. Leave the oil-covered blossoms in a sunny window for two-to-three weeks. The oil turns a deep, brilliant red color as the plant constituents in the blossoms seep into the oil. Strain the oil through cheesecloth, discard the blossoms and store the oil in the refrigerator.

Saint John's Wort oil is a wonderful remedy for nerve pain and burns. Remember, though, that applying oil to a burn will increase the intensity of the burn. Wait until the late stages of burn recovery to use St. John's Wort *oil*. St. John's Wort *gel*, or simply the crushed flowers, would be more appropriate in the early stages of recovering from a burn.

Concentrated Gemmotherapy remedies are made from the buds, young shoots and young rootlets of plants. These buds and shoots have enormous concentrations of nutrients, enzymes and hormonal substances to catalyze the next season's growth. The buds or shoots are macerated (mashed) with 50 percent alcohol, 30 percent glycerin and 20 percent water.

The first herbalists to prepare and use these "embryonic" parts of the plant were in ancient Egypt. Gemmotherapy was rediscovered and researched in Europe over the last century. In the last two decades, Gemmotherapy has become more widely known and practiced in North America.

HOMEOPATHIC REMEDIES

Modern homeopathic medicine is based on the rediscovery of an ancient principle, using like to treat like. Developed by Dr. Samuel Hahnemann, a late 18th century physician, this form of medicine aims to stimulate the body's innate healing capacity to bring about a "cure." The science of homeopathy grew out of Hahnemann's years of medical-text translations. Discouraged by the medical practices of his day, Hahnemann abandoned his medical practice and translated medical texts to support his large family. He also hoped to discover universal laws of healing that were more effective than the conventional medicine of his day, which relied on bleeding, blistering, herbs, sulfur and petroleum for its cures.

While translating *Cullen's Material Medica,* Hahnemann noted Cullen's explanation for why quinine effectively treated malaria. The author hypothesized that quinine treated malaria because of its astringent properties. To test this idea, Hahnemann took four drams (one-half ounce), or about 15 doses, of quinine every morning and evening. Within four days he *developed* the symptoms of malaria in his formerly healthy body. When Hahnemann stopped taking the quinine, the malaria symptoms resolved.

With this experiment, Hahnemann confirmed "the Law of Similars," using like to treat like. In other words, a substance that produced symptoms in a healthy person can be used in dilute form to treat the same symptoms in an ailing person.

Hahnemann and his students tested many substances to discover their effects on a healthy person. They would take careful notes about all of the changes that the remedy would produce, e.g., new physical symptoms, food cravings, sleep position, mood changes, sleep patterns, etc. Each person would take careful notes about the changes he or she experienced. These individual notes would be compiled to create a composite picture of the effects of the remedy. If a symptom or physical change commonly occurred, this symptom was called a "keynote" for the remedy. These research studies of particular substances are called "provings," e.g., proving the effect of a substance on a healthy body.

During his years of research, Hahnemann discovered another basic truth: The more dilute the medicine, the more potent its effect. His discovery ran contrary to the practices of his day, an era when doctors prescribed large doses of mercury, sulfur, coal oil and other toxic substances to produce violent, cathartic effects in the body.

A patient recently reported that a national news program had conducted an exposé on homeopathic medicine. "The reporters discovered there wasn't anything in the remedies!" said the patient, certain that he had debunked any possible claims about homeopathy's effectiveness.

"The reporter was absolutely correct," I replied, smiling patiently. "Beyond a 12c potency of a remedy, there is no physical matter in the remedy. What the reporter didn't talk about, though, was that research in Germany shows that whatever substance was used to prepare the remedy is imprinted in the molecular structure of the water, and that imprint grows stronger with each dilution."

The patient looked mystified. We talked about water's ability to imprint anything it comes in contact with. This understanding of water's miraculous physical properties has been popularized by the Japanese scientist Masaru Emoto. His book, *Hidden Messages in Water* (Beyond Words Publishing, Inc., 2004), beautifully illustrates how water literally carries the imprint of both gross and subtle contacts.

"But is homeopathy scientific?" the man asked. "I mean, if you can't measure any substance in the medicine, is there any scientific basis for these medicines?"

"Homeopathy is definitely scientific," I replied. "In fact, it is one of the purest sciences I have ever studied. Homeopathy relies on the very foundations of Western scientific research: Set an experiment in motion—in this case, taking large doses of a particular substance—and then meticulously observe the effects. That's what Hahnemann and his students and now contemporary homeopathic researchers are doing when they 'prove' a remedy.

"With the development of the electron microscope," I explained, "we were actually able to see the effect of the homeopathic dilutions on the molecular structure of the water. German researchers used this new technology, the electron microscope, to demonstrate that the imprint of the substance on the molecular structure of the water increases with each dilution. That's why the more dilute the remedy is, the greater its effect."

The patient looked doubtful. I smiled again.

"I know this is hard for many people to understand or accept," I said. "This is just the opposite of what the conventional pharmaceutical world teaches."

Remember the spectrum of medicine presented earlier, which ranges from charcoal to diamond? Different assumptions and "laws" are in play at different ends of the spectrum. These laws do not invalidate each other; they are simply describing radically different processes in the body. The two ends of the spectrum require different paradigms and different measuring devices to explain their effects.

Some researchers claim homeopathy is not scientific because it is not easily tested using the current double-blind, placebo-controlled study method of testing pharmaceutical medications. Homeopathy does not fit neatly into that model because it is a medicine that is prescribed for a particular *person*, not the disease he or she is suffering with. I might have 10 people with eczema, for example, and send them home with 10 different remedies. I would be prescribing a remedy for that particular person, based on their individual symptoms.

In contrast, the double-blind, placebo-controlled study would require me to give each person the same remedy. That completely flies in the face of how homeopathic remedies are prescribed. In this case, the measuring tool is not effective for the object or method. Imagine testing the pitch of a musical note using a ruler. The testing device is not appropriate to the phenomenon being measured.

Chinese medicine shares a similar conundrum, which we will discuss in more detail below. Because Chinese medicine views the entire constellation of symptoms a patient is experiencing and then creates a "symptom picture," the double-blind, placebo-controlled study method also does not accurately match the system being studied. Instead of mass trials as a foundation for Chinese medicine, the practitioners study particular cases and, from these cases, learn to apply the methodology of seeing a complete, complex picture to their own patients.

Ways to learn homeopathic remedies

Homeopathic practitioners prescribe either acute or constitutional remedies. Acute remedies address sunburns, colds, bruises or other short-term illnesses. Constitutional remedies treat the big, broad picture of a person—physical symptoms, likes and dislikes, mental attitudes and emotional disposition. Constitutional homeopathy works with the understanding that each of us is layered like an onion. We are born with a particular core, constitutional remedy type. Over time, both positive and negative experiences add layers to that core, so that eventually we are layered like an onion.

When I am prescribing constitutional homeopathic remedies, I look for the most obvious, external layer and prescribe that remedy. Sometimes I can already see additional, deeper layers, like a palimpsest, with other remedies "bleeding through" into the top layer of remedies. In ancient Mesopotamia, people scraped and then reused papyrus reed tablets for writing. Often the reader could discern the fainter, deeper carving of an earlier writer. This "palimpsest," or traces of an earlier scribe, are like the deeper layers of constitutional homeopathic remedies: They are visible as faint etchings "underneath" the most obvious, topmost remedy.

A constitutional remedy sometimes will cut right through to the "core" of the onion. More commonly, the remedy addresses one layer, which resolves or "peels away;" then, another layer emerges. Constitutional homeopathy usually continues over several years before someone reaches their core remedy.

I give this background about constitutional prescribing so that you understand that the acute homeopathic prescriptions we will be discussing are the highlights, or the "tip of the iceberg," of a constitutional remedy. The complete picture of a remedy is the iceberg; the acute symptoms are its tip. The "flavor" of the complete picture permeates the acute picture but is not completely obvious.

When you buy a homeopathic remedy, or you examine the remedies in your homeopathic kit, you will see one or two conditions mentioned on the tube or bottle. Keep in mind this is only a sliver of the tip of the iceberg.

Recently, when a patient severely burned her leg with boiling water, I recommended she take *Causticum* and *Cantharis,* both classic remedies for second- and third-degree burns. When her husband went to the health food store, he was confused about my prescription because the blue tube had "burning urination" as the primary symptom.

I understand why homeopathic companies put these cryptic descriptions on the bottles; they want to give people some clue about the effects of a remedy. These simplistic descriptions, however, cloud people's ability to understand how to choose homeopathic remedies. These shorthand descriptions fuel the "take this for that" approach most people take in choosing medicines. Homeopathic remedies are more complex; they often have multiple applications.

You have to understand the character, or the "personality," of a remedy to begin to use it correctly.

Imagine that you are getting to know a new classroom, a new group of friends. As you converse with each other, you will discover many facets of this "person's" behavior, character and personality. Please be open to these surprises and don't expect the remedy to have a narrow, monolithic range of actions.

The constitutional remedy includes the big, broad picture of all of the many ways a particular remedy can affect the body, mind and spirit. The acute applications of the remedies that we will be discussing carry the *flavor* of the constitutional picture. In acute situations, you may have only one or two keynotes to guide you. Remember that "keynotes" are the most common symptoms associated with a remedy. Aim for these keynotes, the *Gestalt* of the remedy, when you are choosing an acute prescription.

As you learn the remedies, think of particular situations when you would have used them. Think also of people you know, or aspects of yourself, that remind you of the remedy. These are friends you will be getting better acquainted with, hopefully over many years. Approach them as acquaintances you are eager to know more deeply.

The more time you invest in looking at situations in this way—assessing them for homeopathic remedies—the more easily you will discern the remedy patterns, or multidimensional pictures.

From now on, think about what homeopathic remedies you would use in a particular situation. Maybe you are watching a television program, or listening to a friend describe her child's illness. Think about what remedy might be appropriate in that situation. Even if you do not use the remedy in that particular circumstance, you are developing the "muscle" to think in this way. You will come to know the remedy patterns, the multidimensional "pictures" that describe their effect on the body.

Another aspect of homeopathy I have come to appreciate is that you do not need to search for an explanation for why a symptom is occurring. Someone with a cough, for example, may feel better kneeling on the floor with his or her head on the ground. Instead of asking, "Why are they doing *that*? How could that be helping your cough?," you can run to a homeopathic *materia medica* and look up that particular "strange, rare and peculiar symptom." These unusual symptoms can help guide you to the correct remedy.

Homeopathic *materia medicas* represent an advanced aspect of prescribing homeopathic remedies; this is part of coming to know your new acquaintances at much deeper, more intimate levels. The *materia medicas* are indexes of symptoms, arranged by body parts, organs, glands and systems. Each entry, or "rubric," lists homeopathic remedies that will address a particular symptom. In constitutional prescribing, you might look up several rubrics and then cross-reference the remedies that are common to all of the rubrics. This is a very advanced stage of homeopathic prescribing. See the Appendices for a list of commonly used homeopathic *materia medicas*.

How homeopathic medicines are made

Homeopathic remedies are made in "x," "c," "k," and "m" potencies. These numbers describe the potency, or the level of dilution, used to make a remedy. Remember that, in homeopathy, the higher the number, the more dilute the substance.

X potencies are diluted 1:10. One drop of a "mother tincture," prepared from the whole plant, is diluted in *10 drops of water* and then secussed to make a 1x potency. "Secussing" means to bang the closed container against your palm or another cushioned surface. This action "potentizes" the water. In other words, secussing transfers an imprint of the substance to the water's molecular structure. One drop from that dilution is placed in another 10 drops of water and secussed again to make a 2x potency. The dilutions continue until you arrive at the desired dose. Common "x" potencies include 3x, 6x, 30x and 200x. A 30x potency would be 10-to-the-30th power diluted. In other words, the dilutions are *exponential*, not additive.

C and K potencies are both dilutions with 100 drops of water. The remedies are prepared in the same way, adding one drop of mother tincture, in this case, to *100 drops of water*. The remedy is seccussed, then one drop is added to another 100 drops of water. Common dilutions are 6c (or 6k), 12c, 30c and 200c. The highest potency remedies health food stores are allowed to stock is 30c potency. You must buy higher potencies (e.g., 200c) from a trained health care practitioner.

M potencies are diluted with 1,000 drops of water. Common dilutions include 1M, 10M and 50M dilutions. These extremely high potencies are also available only through health care practitioners.

How to care for homeopathic remedies

- Store remedies away from mint, menthol, camphor and perfumes. Because homeopathic remedies are so dilute and, therefore, "subtle," they are susceptible to being "antidoted" by strong-smelling substances.
- Store homeopathic remedies away from essential oils, even those that are not mint or camphor-based. The essential oils can also overpower the homeopathic remedies.
- Store in a cool, dark area. Excessive heat can also destroy the active principles of the remedy.
- If stored in a cool, dry area away from strong-smelling substances, these homeopathic medicines can last for years or even decades.

NOTE: If you are in an emergency situation and have a remedy but are afraid that the remedy is too old or has been "antidoted," go ahead and give the remedy anyhow. Sometimes the remedy will work, even in the worst of circumstance. One of my mentors told the story of traveling with his son in the car. He had a family homeopathic kit in the front seat that had been exposed to lots of summer sun and heat; the bottles were scattered all around the passenger floor in the front seat. His son had a peppermint in his mouth. Despite all of these "red flags," he gave his son the remedy (Apis, for a bee sting), which worked beautifully. If in doubt, give the remedy. The worst it can do is nothing.

How to take homeopathic remedies

The "art" of taking homeopathic remedies involves choosing the correct potency of the remedy and knowing how often to repeat a dose. This form of medication requires a very different awareness of the body and its responses than conventional prescription medicines that are dosed by rote: Take one tablet twice a day with food. Occasionally homeopathic remedies are prescribed on a similar schedule. For acute prescribing, however, you will need to watch the body and its response to the remedy to decide when and if to repeat another dose.

Homeopathy requires your observation and participation to dose correctly. This mindful observation strengthens our connection with and understanding of the body. This medicine roots us more firmly in our bodies, instead of encouraging us to abdicate our connection with our physical form.

General rules of thumb for acute prescribing

During an acute illness, wait at least two hours before deciding if the remedy has helped. By "helped," I do *not* mean that the symptoms have completely resolved. If you were coughing every two minutes and now you are coughing every 10 minutes, then that is a significant improvement. Wait until the coughing worsens—e.g., you are coughing every six or seven minutes—before you repeat the remedy again.

In extremely acute cases, you might be dosing a remedy every 15 minutes. As the pain and inflammation resolve, reduce the frequency of the dosing.

After a car crash, for example, you might be dosing homeopathic Arnica every 15 minutes for the first two hours. As symptoms of shock pass, you might take a dose every hour. The next day, awakening with a stiff neck and general bruising, you likely would continue dosing every hour or two. The second day after the accident, you might be taking a dose every two to three hours. That dose might continue for a week or more, until you reach another plateau in the healing process, at which time you would reduce the frequency to every four or five hours. Continue taking the remedy, at less and less frequent intervals, until the condition has resolved or until the symptom picture changes.

Within one episode of a cold, for example, you might progress through two or even three remedies. This example will make more sense after you have studied the remedies for cold and flu. Imagine that you begin a cold with a sudden, high fever. You are glassy-eyed, with a hot, red face. You have nightmares with the high fever. At this beginning stage, the appropriate remedy would be homeopathic Belladonna.

If the cold does not resolve in this early stage, but progresses to nasal congestion and a rumbling cough, with lots of thick, green mucous discharge, you are ready for a different remedy. The symptom picture has changed. If you feel better outside and long to have someone to cuddle with, you likely need the homeopathic remedy Pulsatilla.

Let's imagine the "cold" moves into the ears and you develop a severe ear infection. Your ears are exquisitely sensitive; the smallest draft of air causes excruciating pain. You have a scarf around your head, even while inside. Your throat is sore with a sticking sensation, as if a fish bone was lodged in the throat. Now you are in need of homeopathic Hepar sulphuricum calcareum, or "Hepar sulph" for short.

In this one example, you can see that the remedy changes as the symptoms change. In addition, the remedies likely will vary from illness to illness. Just because you needed Belladonna, Pulsatilla and Hepar sulph for *this* particular illness does NOT mean that these will be the required remedies for a future respiratory tract infection.

Potency

Another factor to consider in prescribing homeopathic remedies is the potency you choose. In health food stores, you will have access to both x and c potencies. The following guidelines can help you navigate which potency to choose. Understand that some of the principles are contradictory. This is the ART in prescribing homeopathics. You will develop a feel for which remedy and which potency to choose over time, with practice.

- The more acute (brief and severe) the symptoms, the higher the potency and the more frequent the dose.
- The more severe the symptoms, the higher the potency and the more frequent the dose.
- The greater the overlap between the remedy picture and the symptoms the patient is presenting, the higher the potency.
- The more physical the symptoms, the *lower* the potency.
- The more mental or emotional the symptoms, the *higher* the potency.
- The higher the potency, the less frequently you will need to dose.

I understand some of the guidelines are contradictory. What if you have great overlap between the symptom picture and the patient (give a high potency), but he or she has primarily physical symptoms (give low potency)? You have a couple of choices. You can give the high potency remedy and watch for results. If you wait an hour or two and have no response, move to the lower potency.

Of course, you may have only one potency available. If you have only one potency, give the remedy and watch the body's response. Repeat the remedy as needed.

When I was in a major car wreck, for example, I had my trusty homeopathic travel kit in the back seat. I immediately took my backpack with the remedies out of the crushed car and began dosing Arnica 30c (classic for trauma, bruising, hemorrhage and shock), which I consider to be a "mid-range" potency. I began taking a dose of Arnica 30c every five-to-10 minutes for the first hour, then every 15-to-30 minutes for the next three or four hours.

When I got home after the accident, which took place about 200 miles from home, I had access to higher potency remedies. That first night I took an extremely high dose of Arnica—50 M. I repeated that dose the next morning and two or three times later in the day. Notice that, with the higher dose, I reduced the frequency of dosing.

The second day after the accident, I chose a 1M potency of Arnica. I continued taking the 1M Arnica three or four times a day. After another few days, I reduced the potency to 200c. I continued dosing this potency three or four times a day for the next two weeks, until most of the deep bruises in my legs had resolved.

In this example, I was changing the potency as well as the frequency of the dose, depending on the severity of the injury and where I was in the healing process. As my symptoms improved, I reduced the potency as well as the frequency of dosing. I knew the remedy helped because when the colleague who treated my injuries looked at the picture of the totaled car and then looked at me, she gave a low whistle.

"I can't believe how little bruising you have with this level of damage to the car," she said. "That's amazing!"

I still had deep bruises covering much of my body, but my colleague, who had treated many motor vehicle accident patients, knew how bad the injuries *could* be. She knew from past experience that patients who had endured a similar accident generally had much more trauma and much more bruising.

In most health food stores, the highest potency you will find is a 30c. As mentioned earlier, I consider this to be a mid-range potency. If you have a serious injury or condition, you likely will need to make up for the lower-than-optimal potency by dosing it more frequently. If I had had only the 30c potency after my car wreck, I would have continued taking the remedy more frequently. In my situation, because I had access to high potency remedies, I took the higher potencies less frequently. I reduced the potency, rather than the frequency, as symptoms improved.

You likely will be reducing frequency, rather than the potency of the remedy. In the earlier example, when taking homeopathic Belladonna for a sudden, high fever, you might be taking a dose of the remedy every hour or two. You would repeat a dose when the fever begins to spike again (I'm guessing here; your actual experience, not my estimates, is your best guide.). When you move into a later stage of the cold—e.g., the thick, green mucous stage common for homeopathic Pulsatilla—you might be taking a dose of the remedy two or three times a day.

Children usually respond to lower potencies, e.g., 6c or 12c potencies. Their bodies are vital enough that they often do not need as strong a "catalyst" as the higher potency remedies provide. This also is a general rule of thumb. Sometimes I've given my boys a lower potency of a well-indicated remedy, with little-to-no effect. I've switched to a higher potency and they have responded well. Allow the child's responses to the remedy to guide your decision-making.

Again, you will develop a "feel" for dosing over time. This is the art of homeopathic prescribing. Although later in the book you will see that I give estimates for potency and frequency of dosing, please understand these are ballpark directives. Homeopathy works best when you are actively engaged in observing the body's response to the remedy and dose accordingly. Unlike pharmaceutical drugs that are prescribed on a rote basis, with an unwavering dose no matter how the body is responding, homeopathy requires you to alter the frequency as the body improves so that you *take the remedy only as needed.*

Patients sometimes ask if they can take a homeopathic remedy to *prevent* illness. Only in a couple of rare situations do I recommend "prophylactic" homeopathic remedies. Generally, you take homeopathic remedies *only when the symptoms are present,* not when you *expect* the symptoms to develop. When everyone in the house has a cold and you want to avoid being sick, for example, I would suggest taking botanicals and nutrients to bolster the immune system, rather than taking homeopathic remedies. Save the homeopathic remedies for the onset of symptoms, *if* needed.

ESSENTIAL OILS

These oils are extremely concentrated preparations of a plant's volatile oils. One drop of an essential oil, for example, is roughly equivalent to 30 cups of tea! One ounce of essential oil of rose requires approximately two tons (4,000 pounds) of rose petals. These extremely concentrated plant preparations border on a synthetic substance, because they are such highly concentrated preparations of particular constituents in the plant. Use them with utmost respect.

Skin application

Essential oils are best applied externally, on the skin, diluted with carrier oil. Add one or two drops to a teaspoon of vegetable oil and then apply to the skin. Examples of good vegetable oils for essential oil application include olive, coconut, almond, sesame and avocado. You may discover other vegetable oils you enjoy as well.

The two most absorptive skin surfaces on the body are the palms of the hands and the soles of the feet. You can take advantage of these absorptive surfaces by applying the diluted essential oils in these areas. In the winter, I often rub tea tree essential oil in the bottom of my boys' feet to boost their immune system and address any bacteria and viruses developing in their bodies.

Misting with essential oils

You can also protect your family from cold and flu viruses by preparing an essential oil spray to mist the air. These air mist preparations are also an excellent way to deliver essential oils to improve mood and concentration, as the inhalation of essential oils directly affects brain function. When inhaled, the oils move directly through the nasal passages and into the brain. This characteristic makes essential oils one of the fastest, most effective ways of altering brain chemistry as well as supporting respiratory function.

To prepare a 1% solution of essential oils for misting: in an 8-ounce spray bottle of water, add 48 drops of essential oil. Add one tablespoon of vodka, to help disperse the essential oil in the water. Shake before using.

For a 3% solution, good for combating mosquitoes and other insects, add 144 drops of essential oil to 8 ounces of water. Add a tablespoon of vodka to help disperse the oil in water.

You may choose to use one oil, or a combination of two. While you are learning about essential oils, I would not suggest using more than two oils at a time.

Taking essential oils internally

DO NOT take essential oils internally unless you have had advanced training. Ingesting these extremely concentrated preparations can damage the liver and other organs if you dose incorrectly. Work with a health care provider trained in using essential oils who can guide you in internal use of the essential oils. Please do not rely on someone trained by a multi-level marketing company. Although many of these essential oils are very high quality, their primary goal is to sell essential oils, NOT provide the safest, most effective delivery of their products.

Ways to apply essential oils:

- Skin application
  - Dilution with vegetable oil
  - Hands and feet, especially with children, for systemic effect
- Steam inhalation (close the eyes!)
- Inhaler
- Mist – insect repellant; air freshener/purifier
- Terra cotta figures impregnated with oil
- On a tissue – short-term replacement for inhaler
- AVOID heating essential oils, which oxidizes the oils, causing lung damage
- AVOID ingestion; hard on the liver. You need advanced training to prescribe essential oils for internal use

Essential oils that are safe for children and babies

- Babies: rose, lavender, Roman chamomile. 1/6 adult dosage
- Ages 18 months to 4 years: mandarin, tangerine, tea tree, Eucalyptus radiata (NOT the more common Eucalyptus globulus, which is a stronger, more stimulating oil). ¼ adult dosage
- Ages 5 to 12: spearmint, other citruses (e.g. grapefruit, orange). ½ adult dosage

Safely storing essential oils

- Keep out of the reach of children.
- Keep cap on.
- Store in a cool, dark area.
- Store in brown or deep violet glass bottles; will destroy most plastics and rubber.
- Rebottle when the bottle is less than half full (air oxidizes oil).

FLOWER ESSENCES

The most recent renaissance of flower essences was spurred by the work of Edward Bach, M.D. After Dr. Bach completed his medical training in England in the 1880's, he studied and researched vaccinations. In addition, he studied homeopathy, which was one of the most commonly used forms of medicine in his day. In his practice, he observed that patients tended toward illness when they developed certain mental and emotional patterns. Fascinated with this connection between mental, emotional and physical health, he left his practice in England to return to his native home in Wales.

There he roamed the countryside, walking and looking for plants that drew his attention. Much like the Anishnabe bear/healer story, he would develop a condition and then wander through the lanes and meadows, asking to be drawn to the plant that would heal his illness.

When he found the plant, he would gather the blossoms and prepare them as a "flower essence." Although Bach is credited with the development of flower essences, in truth he was rediscovering an ancient practice of plant preparation. He would place the flowers in a small glass bowl filled with spring water and leave the flower filled bowl of water in the sun for four hours. This water was "potentized" by contact with the flowers and the sun. This "essence" was preserved with alcohol and reserved to make "stock," for further dilutions of the remedy.

> Essence → Stock → Medicine

- Essence = the potentized water, mixed with an equal amount of brandy
- Stock = two drops of essence in 30 ml of pure brandy
- Medicine = two drops of stock in a small bottle (30 ml) of mixed water and brandy (usually two parts water to one part brandy)
- 8 ounces of essence makes millions of doses of medicine!

Over the course of four years, Bach discovered and researched 38 remedies. Those who have studied Bach's work claim that these 38 remedies are the only ones humanity will ever need to address all disease. Bach himself, however, encouraged people to develop their own relationship with plant allies. In his book, *The Seven Healers,* Bach notes that "In this system of healing everything may be done by the people themselves, even, if they like, the finding of the plants and the making of the remedies."

Do you recognize the process of "deep listening" in Bach's work? You can develop your own relationship with particular plants as healing allies. When you are sick or feeling imbalanced, spend time outdoors. Allow yourself to be drawn to the plant or plants that speak to you. Consciously work with these herbal healers and allies. These green allies likely have gifts to offer you, to support you in your healing process.

I have also learned about flower essences from R.J. Stewart, a phenomenally gifted keeper of the ancient Celtic traditions. R.J. gave me a wider historical and cultural context for flower essences. Through him I learned that many cultures around the world have used this method of preparing essence for many generations. R.J. teaches a much older, more traditional method of preparing flower essences that foregoes cutting the flower from the plant to prepare the essence. Cutting the flowers would be a shock and an insult to the plant. Instead, the traditional method of preparing flower essences involved building a support under the plant so that the bowl of water would reach the flowers. This method bypassed the need to cut the flowers.

Please see the Appendices for more detailed instructions for preparing plant essences. I would encourage you to follow the older, more traditional method as much as possible. In my experience, the flower essences are much more potent when prepared without cutting the flowers from the plants.

As mentioned earlier, the primary sphere of influence for the flower essences is the mental emotional realm. The flower essences do not take away emotions or attempt to "cure" them, like anti-depressants or anti-anxiety drugs. Instead, the flower essences provide more ballast so that we can more easily address the emotional issues that face us.

In turn, as the mental and emotional spheres are harmonized, the physical body can relax into a more functional, balanced state. The flower essences can and do have profound effects on the physical body. The avenues through which they reach the physical body are the mental and emotional realms.

One of the best ways to experience the flower essences is to use Rescue Remedy™, a wonderful combination of five flower essences developed specifically for shock and trauma.

The five flowers include:

- Clematis
- Rock Rose
- Impatiens
- Star of Bethlehem
- Cherry Plum

I've provided a brief introduction to these five essences, so that you can begin to get the "flavor" of the remedies and how they work. Notice how each approaches shock and/or trauma from a different direction; each has a different way of offering support.

Clematis vitalba – Clematis
- Dreamy, drowsy, not fully awake, no great interest in life
- In illness, makes little or no effort to get well
- May look forward to death
- Acute – typical of shock
- Deeper presentation – depressed, even suicidal

Helianthemum nummularium - Rock Rose
- Emergency, for cases that appear to have no hope
- THE "rescue remedy," according to Bach
- Accidents, sudden illness, trauma, violence when the person is frightened or terrified
- If unconscious, can moisten the lips with the remedy.
- Can be helpful in the dying process, when someone is afraid, viewing death as total annihilation.
- Name derives from Greek *Helios*, the sun, and the Latin word for coins. Restores sun-like forces of courage to the human soul to meet tremendous challenges.

Impatients glandulifera - Impatiens
- Quick in thought and action
- Wishes everything to be completed without delay
- Difficult to be patient with people who are slow
- Wrong to waste time
- For acute: anxious to recover quickly

Ornitholagum umbellatum - Star of Bethlehem
- Shock of any kind tends to drive us out of our bodies.
- "I jumped out of my skin" or "I was beside myself."
- Shocking news, the loss of a beloved, fright following an accident
- Soothes and comforts, which helps to alleviate pain

- Star of Bethlehem unifies body and soul again so that the natural healing processes can take place.

Prunus cerasifera - Cherry Plum

- Fear of reason giving way, of doing fearful and dreaded things, not wished and known wrong, yet there comes the thought and impulse to do them
- The soul tries to protect against this fear of losing control by tightening its grip, which only leads to more pressure and stress.
- Cherry Plum gives mental strength and confidence.

Consider using Rescue Remedy™ in the following situations:

- Physical trauma
- Before and after dental work
- After shocking news
- Grief
- Insomnia
- Anxiety
- High-stress situations, e.g., before a performance, test, job interview, public speech

HYDROTHERAPY

Earth is a water planet, bestowed with a blue-green vastness of liquid life. Our bodies are 70 percent water—we left the amniotic support of the sea by learning to contain it within our skin. Humans can survive for weeks without food. Without water, we perish within days or even hours in an arid desert climate.

For thousands of years water has been used to treat disease and trauma. In the 19th and 20th centuries, physicians combined these ancient therapies with modern scientific research. At his mountain sanitarium, Vincent Priessnitz (1799-1852) championed the European rediscovery of water's healing properties. In the United States, John Harvey Kellogg, M.D., (1852-1945) was a major proponent of water cures. His Battle Creek Sanitarium combined water treatments with sine-wave, massage and dietary therapies. His method of pressing whole grains into "flakes" survives today in the Kellogg cereal industry. Kellogg kept meticulous records and conducted scientific research in his sanitarium. The data gathered became the foundation for *Rational Hydrotherapy* (F.A. David, 1901), still the definitive textbook on the subject.

Hydrotherapy involves the use of hot and cold water in specific treatments to stimulate the immune system and alter blood circulation to particular areas of the body. Outlined below are six specific hydrotherapy treatments that can be used to treat a wide range of conditions.

GENERAL CAUTION: Diabetic patients must be careful with hot applications to the feet. Most diabetics have reduced nerve sensation in the feet and are more likely to burn the skin by accident. This also applies to anyone with compromised circulation in the extremities (e.g., Raynaud's Syndrome). Have someone else test the water OR apply a large fomentation (towels wrung out in very warm water) to the groin area.

Constitutional Hydrotherapy Treatment

The constitutional hydrotherapy treatment boosts immune function by increasing red-and-white blood cell production and activity; improves digestion; and promotes detoxification. This treatment can be used to treat almost any acute or chronic condition. In a hydrotherapy clinic, the treatment would include a sine-wave machine to further stimulate the digestive tract. The following instructions are for home application. Repeat the treatment once daily.

When not to apply this treatment: in acute cases of asthma or low body temperature (below 97°F oral temperature, unless this is your "normal" temperature). Be careful to avoid drafts or chills during the treatment. Apply a hot water bottle to the feet and add more blankets if you feel chilly.

Self-application method

Supplies:
- Shower or bath
- 2 Blankets (ideally wool)
- 1 Towel
- 1 Sheet

Directions:
- Spread 2 blankets lengthwise on a bed with a sheet over them.
- Wet the towel with cold water and wring out excess water. The towel should be thoroughly wet but not dripping.
- Take a hot bath or shower, as hot as you can comfortably stand, for 5-to-10 minutes. You should feel warm after the bath or shower; if not, postpone the treatment until you are feeling warmer.

- Step out of the shower and dry off.
- Fold the wet towel in half and place it over your chest and abdomen, as illustrated below. Later, when you can easily warm the towel on the front, wrap the towel all the way around your trunk.
- Lie face up on the sheet and blankets you prepared earlier.
- Wrap the sheets and blankets snugly around you.
- Sleep, rest, meditate or listen to quiet music for 25-to-30 minutes, or until your body has warmed the toweling.

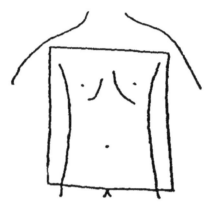

Assisted method (i.e., you have someone to help you)

Supplies:

- Shower or Bath
- 4 towels
- 2 blankets (ideally wool)
- 1 sheet

Directions

1 Spread 2 blankets lengthwise on a bed with the sheet over them.
2 The person being treated lies on his or her back, unclothed from the hips up.
3 Thoroughly wet 2 towels with hot water and place them on the chest and abdomen, as illustrated below. The towel should be wet through, but not dripping

4   Wrap the sheet and blankets tightly around them and leave in place for 5 minutes.

5   Thoroughly wet one towel with cold water. The towel should be wet through, but not dripping.

6   Remove the hot, wet towels and replace them with the cold, wet towel.

7   Wrap the sheet and blankets tightly around the patient.

8   Sleep, rest, meditate or listen to quiet music for at least 10 minutes, or until the towel is warm to the touch.

9   Repeat this procedure with the person lying on his stomach and apply towels to his back. Rest and leave in place for at least 10 minutes.

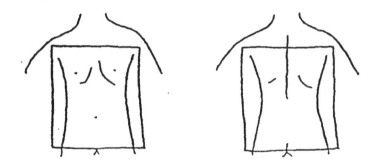

Salt Water Lavage and Gargle

This treatment eliminates excess mucous from the nose and throat. Salt water soothes inflamed tissue and destroys bacteria and viruses. Because the salt solution is more concentrated than the saline inside the bacteria and virus, it literally causes the microbes to explode.

Begin gargling with salt water at the first sign of a sore throat. Repeat every two hours until the symptoms resolve. Use the nasal lavage technique when nasal congestion develops, or after exposure to irritating inhalants (e.g., dust, air pollution, mold).

Equipment

- Tall glass or large cup
- Water, as warm as you can comfortably tolerate
- 1-to-2 teaspoons of sea salt (non-iodized)

Directions

1 Add sea salt to glass of warm water.
2 For gargle, take one mouthful of salt water at a time. Some physicians recommend swallowing the salt water after gargling. Do not swallow the salt water if you have hypertension or diabetes.
3 For nasal lavage, pour salt water into your cupped hand. Gently inhale the salt water and then gently blow the water from the nostrils. This is best done over a sink. At the end of the treatment, be sure to blow any excess water from the nose. You may notice increased nasal and sinus drainage after the treatment.

NOTE: Too much or too little salt or cool water may cause nasal tingling and discomfort. Adjust the water temperature or amount of salt if you experience nasal discomfort.

Neti pot

This cleansing method rinses the nasal-sinus passages with warm salt water. The neti pot is calibrated to control the amount of water flowing from the pot to deliver a steady, gentle stream of salt water to cleanse away dust, pollen and/or mold. The neti pot can also be used during an acute cold or sinus infection to help rinse away the accumulated mucous and deliver saline solution and herbs directly into the nasal-sinus area.

Equipment

• Neti pot
• Warm water
• Sea salt

Optional: essential oil, hydrogen peroxide, special herbal combinations

Directions

1 Fill the neti pot with wrist-warm water.
2 Add the amount of salt recommended in the neti pot instructions. Be sure to use the recommended amount of salt. Either too little or too much salt will cause burning in the nose. The recommended amount of salt will yield an isotonic solution, the same salinity as our own bodies.
3 Bend forward over the sink and tip your head to one side.

4   Place the neti pot in the upper nostril and allow the saline solution to flow in the upper nostril and out the lower nostril.

5   When you have used the entire pot, breathe out strongly through both open nostrils. If you close one nostril when you breathe out, you will create a backpressure that will cause the saline to move into the sinuses and possibly the ears. Leaving both nostrils open is just the opposite of what most of us were instructed to do as children!

6   Refill the neti pot and rinse the nostrils from the other side.

Optional: You can add other medicinals to the neti pot. During an acute cold, you can add one drop of tea tree essential oil to combat the viral and/or bacterial infection. I emphasize *one drop* because essential oils are extremely potent. Remember that one drop of an essential oil is roughly equivalent to 30 cups of tea.

Hydrogen peroxide can also help resolve nasal and sinus infections. Carefully measure and add one teaspoon of hydrogen peroxide to the neti pot each time you refill it. *Add hydrogen peroxide in addition to the salt.* The hydrogen peroxide does *not* substitute for the salt.

Himalaya Institute makes two different types of Neti Wash that you also can add to the neti pot. One contains zinc, a mineral known to increase immune system activity, as well as herbs. The second formulation includes essential oils and herbs, but no zinc.

During peak allergy season, you can use the neti pot three or four times a day. The neti rinse will help reduce the pollen load in the nostrils.

You may also choose to use the neti pot two or three times a day during an acute cold. If your nasal passages are extremely swollen, you may have to wait for several seconds before the saline begins to move through the nasal passages. I usually wait up to one minute; if no salt water passes through, I try tipping my head in the opposite direction and waiting for up to another minute. Usually the congestion will begin to break up if you are patient and wait a few seconds. Very occasionally, the nostrils are simply too swollen to allow the passage of the salt water. If the nostrils are too plugged or too inflamed, wait an hour or two and try again. Inhaling steam before using the neti pot may help to open the nasal passages.

Wet-Socks Treatment

This simple, powerful treatment stimulates the production and activity of white blood cells and draws congestion away from the upper body. The wet-socks treatment speeds resolution of an upper-respiratory infection. If used when the very first symptoms begin, the treatment can even abort a cold.

Equipment

- Foot bath (a plastic dishpan works well, or sit on the edge of a bathtub and soak feet in hot, shallow water)
- Towel
- 1 pair of cotton ankle-high socks
- 1 pair of wool socks

Directions

1. Soak feet in water as hot as you can comfortably tolerate for 5-to-10 minutes. Add more hot water if necessary.
2. Dry feet.
3. Wet cotton socks in cold tap water. Wring out thoroughly. Socks should be damp, not dripping.
4. Get in bed. Put on the damp cotton socks. Immediately cover with the wool socks.
5. Go to sleep.

NOTE: This treatment is best done right before bedtime. In most cases, the socks will be dry by morning.

Hot Foot Bath

A hot foot bath can treat a wide variety of ailments, from simple tension headaches, to upper-respiratory infections and menstrual cramps.

Equipment

- Plastic dishpan, tub, or bowl large enough to soak the feet
- Towel for drying feet

Directions

1. Fill the pan with enough water to cover the ankles. The water should be as hot as you can comfortably stand it.
2. Soak the feet for 5-to-10 minutes maximum. More than 10 minutes of heat exposure promotes congestion more than circulation.

For a more powerful treatment, alternate between hot-water and cold-water baths.

1   Soak the feet in hot water for 5 minutes.
2   Soak the feet in cold water for 1 minute.
3   Repeat this cycle at least 3 times.
4   Always end with cold water.

Alternating Hot and Cold Applications

Alternating hot and cold applications to a local area increases circulation and decreases congestion. From a Chinese perspective, congestion or "stagnation" causes pain. This simple method can be employed to reduce pain and swelling associated with acute injuries, ear infections, headaches and other conditions.

In general, the greater the contrast in temperature between the hot and cold applications, the stronger is the effect of the treatment. For children, the elderly and severely debilitated people (e.g., terminal cancer, late stages of AIDS, or emphysema), moderate the temperature extremes.

Equipment

- 2 towels
- A large pan of hot water, or a microwave
- A pan of cold water, with ice cubes (if tolerated)
- Plastic sheet (or an old shower curtain), if needed to protect bedding

Directions

1   Always begin with a 3-to-5-minute hot application. This can be a towel wrung out in hot water (as hot as you can stand it) or a wetted towel placed in a microwave for three to four minutes. If the towel is too hot, shake it back and forth for a couple of moments—towels cool quickly. Apply the towel to the affected area.
2   Apply a cold application (towel wrung out in cold tap water or ice water) to the affected area for 1 minute.
3   Repeat this cycle at least 3 times.
4   Always end with a cold application.

General Advice

- Make sure an area is warm before applying a cold towel. If someone is severely chilled, or if the body temperature is below 98°F, warm the body with a hot bath or shower before applying cold towels.

- For acute earaches, a 40-watt lightbulb can be substituted for a hot, wet towel. Sit 6-to-8 inches away from the lightbulb, close enough to feel heat, but not close enough to burn the skin. To reduce pain associated with earache, use heat alone for up to 30 minutes.
- A hot-water bottle can substitute for a hot, wet towel.
- For a small area, frozen peas in a plastic bag can be substituted for a cold, wet towel.

CASTOR OIL PACKS

When I mention castor oil packs, many patients grimace. They are familiar with taking castor oil by mouth. Used internally, castor oil is a cathartic, meaning it triggers intestinal dumping by irritating the intestines. When used *externally*, however, castor oil can decrease inflammation and soften scar tissue. Generally you will need to repeat the treatment several times, e.g., at least three times a week for a period of time, to reverse chronic inflammation and scar tissue formation.

Equipment

- 1 yard of cotton or wool flannel
- 4 ounces of organic castor oil
- A plastic covering, e.g., a shopping bag
- Hot water bottle or microwave hot pack.

Directions

1 Wash and dry the wool or cotton flannel.
2 Saturate the cloth with castor oil. The cloth should be damp through but not dripping with oil.
3 Place the cloth over the area you are treating.
4 Cover the cloth with plastic to prevent the oil from penetrating clothing, bedding, furniture, etc.
5 Place a hot water bottle or heating pad over the castor oil pack.
6 Rest for 45-to-60 minutes.
7 Store the castor oil pack in a Ziploc® bag or wide-mouthed canning jar in the refrigerator.
8 Before using the pack again, warm *briefly* in the microwave or in a conventional oven (in a metal or glass container). Obviously, heating the pack too long could cause a fire.

9   For subsequent treatments, add additional castor oil to the cloth
     as needed. Remember that the cloth should be saturated, but not
     dripping, with castor oil.

Alternate method: For sore joints, you may choose to apply the castor oil pack
at bedtime and secure with an ACE bandage. Place a towel under the area
being treated, to prevent oil from staining the bedclothes. Leave on overnight
without heat.

You can reuse the castor oil pack 25-to-30 times before washing. Soak the
cloth in baking soda to cut the oil, then wash and dry. You can reapply castor
oil and use the cloth again.

SKIN BRUSHING

Gently brushing the skin removes the surface layer of dead skin cells. Sloughing off this
layer stimulates the body to more effectively discharge waste material through the skin.

Skin brushing also stimulates the lymphatic system, the back-up circulatory
system that parallels our bloodstream. The lymph vessels carry waste and also
ferry immune cells throughout the body.

Equipment

- A textured washcloth
- Loofah
- Vegetable fiber skin brush

Directions:

1   Choose one of the items above. Initially, you probably will want
     to use the washcloth. Eventually, you may progress to a loofah or
     vegetable fiber brush, which has a deeper-acting effect on the skin.
2   Brush gently. Aim to remove only the very superficial layer, not to
     cause bleeding.
3   Always brush toward the heart, the same direction the blood and
     lymph move.
4   Begin at the feet and move upward.
5   Brush only the hairier, "tougher" skin areas. Avoid brushing the softer
     areas, e.g., the belly, particularly with the rougher vegetable fiber brush.
6   Shower or bathe after brushing the skin.

SALT GLOW TREATMENT

The salt glow treatment has a similar effect on the body as skin brushing, removing dead skin cells and stimulating the lymph and blood circulation. In addition, salt supports waste removal through the skin.

Equipment

- Sea salt
- A bowl or basin
- A small bowl of water

Directions

1   Pour sea salt in the bowl
2   Fill your palm with salt and then add a few drops of water.
3   Begin with your feet, rubbing the salt into the soles of the feet.
4   Gradually move up the body, massaging the salt into the skin with a gentle, circling motion.
5   When you have completely massaged the body with salt, step in the shower and rinse off the salt.

ACUPRESSURE

Acupressure means applying gentle, steady pressure to stimulate acupuncture points. Stimulating the points with a needle (acupuncture) generally produces a stronger reaction, yet acupressure still can deeply affect the body without penetrating the skin.

Often acupressure points will feel a bit sore, boggy or "congested." Hold the point with steady pressure for 10-to-30 seconds. You can also "plant" a thumb or finger at the point and then make gentle circles. You will get a feel for how best to stimulate the points over time.

The more relaxed your hand or finger is, the deeper you can penetrate the area without causing pain or bruising.

If an area is already bruised or the skin is damaged (e.g., cut or burned), do NOT use acupressure in that area. For bruised or injured areas, treat the opposite side. For a broken right arm, for example, treat the left arm or the opposite-opposite limb—in this case, the left leg.

Gallbladder 20 (GB 20) is located just below the occipital bone (back of the head), in the hollow behind the trapezius muscle. This point is excellent for the beginning of a cold with runny nose and fever; head pain; headache; neck stiffness; arthritis in the neck and shoulders.

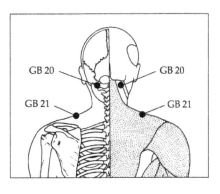

Gallbladder 21 (GB 21) is located on the highest point of the shoulder, 1 – 2 inches from the side of the neck. This point helps lower blood pressure, relieves neck and shoulder tension, reduces nervousness and anxiety, and supports milk production for mothers who are breastfeeding. In general this point has a "down-bearing" effect.

Kidney 1 (K11) is located on the sole of the foot, just behind the ball of the foot. This point is excellent for kidney and bladder issues as well as for emergency conditions, e.g., when someone is losing consciousness. This point is one of the five "mouths of *qi*," or points where the body both absorbs and excretes a tremendous amount of *qi* or vitality. Regularly massaging this point helps to relax the foot, making it easier to absorb *qi* from the Earth.

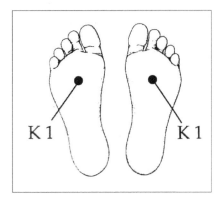

Large Intestine 4 (LI4) is located in the web between the thumb and first finger. The point name *He gu* means "big mouth," probably because this webbed area in the hand looks like a mouth. This point is also known as the ruler of the face and neck and has a profound impact on all conditions in the face and front of the neck, e.g., nasal congestion, headaches and sore throat. This point is used for dental anesthesia, with electrical stimulation.

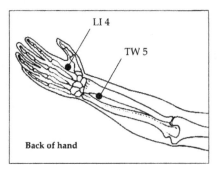

Triple warmer 5 (TW5) is located on the posterior side of the forearm, about 2-to-3 inches above the wrist. This point can be used to treat neck and shoulder pain, headaches, fevers, hand and finger pain and pain in the abdominal region.

Liver 3 (LV3) is located in the web between the first and second toes. This major liver point can be stimulated to ease headaches, eye pain, depression, upper abdominal pain and uterine bleeding. The liver is responsible for smooth circulation of the blood, so stimulating this point aids the liver in smoothly circulating blood throughout the body.

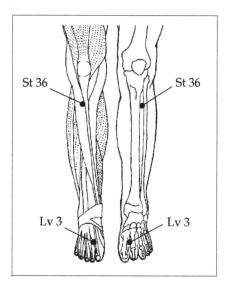

Stomach 36 (ST36) is located just below the *lateral* aspect of the knee. This powerful point addresses stomach pain, vomiting, diarrhea, rumbling in the intestines, constipation, indigestion and knee pain. ST36 may also have some immune-boosting activity for chronic immune deficiency conditions.

Pericardium 6 (PC6) is located on the medial aspect of the forearm, between two tendons, approximately 2-to-3 inches above the wrist (the exact location varies with each person's anatomy). This point soothes the abdomen and chest, addressing nausea and vomiting, abdominal pain, chest pain and heart palpitations. You can buy special bracelets that stimulate this point to treat motion sickness and the nausea of pregnancy.

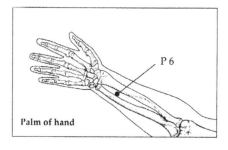

Spleen 6 (SP6) is located one hand-breadth above the medial ankle. All three yin channels on the leg—kidney, spleen and liver—cross at this point, giving rise to the name *San yin jiao*, or "three yin crossing." This point both moves and nourishes blood, making it

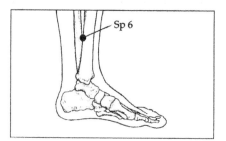

an excellent point for treating what the Chinese refer to as blood and yin deficiency conditions, e.g., menstrual difficulties, abdominal pain, hot flashes, diarrhea, impotence and insomnia.

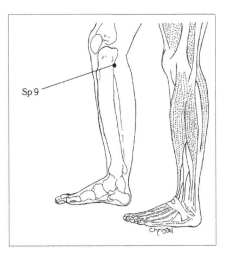

Spleen 9 (SP9) is located just below the *medial* aspect of the knee. This point, like Spleen 6, has a profound effect on the digestive tract and can help ease diarrhea, abdominal bloating and distension and abdominal pain. Stimulating SP9 regulates fluid metabolism and reduces fluid retention and mucous formation. This point also reduces knee pain.

BREATHING EXERCISES

Breath is as much a nutrient as an apple or a piece of toast. Because we do not have to think about breathing (the breath is regulated by the autonomic nervous system), we often forget about the importance of air as a nutrient.

In the last two decades, our knowledge of oxygen intake has advanced to include an understanding that nocturnal lapses in air intake can cause severe problems. Reduced air intake, or "sleep apnea," can reduce oxygen levels in the blood and, therefore, compromise the metabolism in every cell of the body. Many people now sleep with supplemental oxygen to improve their oxygen intake through the night.

Even during the day, many of us breathe shallowly or sometimes hold our breath. When I am concentrating deeply on a project, I may "come to" an hour or more later, hunched over a sewing project or my computer, barely breathing. Although I may not have low oxygen levels, the quality of air in my lungs is certainly diminished, with stale air in the bottom lobes of the lungs.

One of the fastest, most effective ways to increase oxygen levels and stimulate a relaxation response in the body is to breathe deeply. Breathe all the way down to the pubic area. Many of us engage only the chest muscles, and nothing below the diaphragm, when we breathe. Shallow breathing does not have the same rejuvenating, relaxing effect as deep breaths that fill the entire trunk of the body.

Women especially seem to have difficulty allowing the abdomen to expand during an inhalation. Likely, our early training to "suck in the stomach" contributes to this dysfunctional breathing pattern.

Breathing practice

One of the simplest, most enjoyable ways to deepen your breathing is to find a "belly rock," a smooth, rounded rock a little larger than your fist that follows the contours of your belly. I found mine near a river; a beach would be another good place to look.

Lie down with the smooth rock on your belly. How does your body feel? Are certain areas tense or relaxed? Where do you feel heat or coolness in the body?

Next, place your attention on the smooth, rounded surface of the rock. Allow breath to move into the belly and gently push the rock upward. Fill the lower abdomen first; then, allow the upper belly and chest to expand.

When you exhale, allow your lower belly to deflate first, then the upper belly and finally the chest.

On the next inhale, allow the lower belly to rise first. Feel the breath rise, like a fluid wave, through the upper abdomen and into the chest. Sense that wave cresting and then ebbing as the air leaves the lower abdomen, upper abdomen and chest.

Continue this mindful breathing for another three-to-five minutes. Bring your attention back to your body. How do the muscles feel now? Are certain areas looser or tighter than before you started? Do you notice a change in heat or coolness in the body? Observe what, if anything, has changed and then carry on with your day.

This simple exercise can shift your stress levels faster than almost any other relaxation technique. Keep your belly rock in a place where you can easily access it—perhaps one at home and one at work. After awhile you will no longer need the rock, because you can place your attention in the lower abdomen without its gentle, guiding presence.

Alternate nostril breathing

The body naturally shifts the dominant nostril about every two hours. The flow of air, for example, will be stronger in the right nostril from noon to 2 p.m.; then, the air flow will increase in the left nostril.

Speeding the natural alternation of dominant nostrils gently energizes the body, improves circulation, increases relaxation, promotes more restful sleep, calms the nervous system and improves brain function.

Sit in a comfortable position and block the right nostril with your right thumb. Inhale through the open left nostril to a count of four: "One, one-thousand; two, one-thousand; three, one-thousand; four, one-thousand." Count silently to yourself.

Breathe in as smoothly and deeply as you can during these four counts. When you reach the peak of the inhalation, close the left nostril with your index finger. At this point, both nostrils are gently pinched closed. Hold for a count of two.

Release the right thumb and exhale through the right nostril for a count of four: "One, one-thousand; two, one-thousand; three, one-thousand; four, one-thousand." Completely exhale the breath.

At the end of the exhalation, hold both nostrils closed for a count of two.

Open the right nostril again and inhale to the count of four. You are beginning a second complete cycle of alternate nostril breathing.

Begin with three-to-five rounds of alternate nostril breathing. As you become more adept at this breathing technique, you may want to cycle through 10 or more rounds. Over time you can also increase the count for each cycle; e.g., inhale for a count of eight, hold for a count of four, exhale to a count of eight, and hold at the end of the exhale for a count of four.

Lion's Breath

This breathing technique helps completely expel stale air from the base of the lungs. In addition, the Lion's Breath increases circulation in the throat, which can help quell the onset of a sore throat.

Sit cross-legged, or on a chair, if sitting cross-legged is too strenuous. Place your palms face-down on your knees. Breathe in deeply, filling first the abdomen and then the chest. Fill the lungs until you feel they can't hold any more air. Then take three more small "sips" of air.

Exhale sharply as you lean forward and stick out your tongue. Splay your fingers on your knees. The air will "roar" from your lungs. Continue to exhale until no air is left in the lungs.

After you have exhaled as much as you possibly can, relax, sit upright, and allow the air to refill your lungs. Take three deep breaths.

Repeat two more rounds of The Lion's Breath.

This exercise is fantastic for clearing and revitalizing the lungs. I know of several ex-smokers who have tasted cigarette smoke when they practiced the Lion's Breath, sometimes even years after they had stopped smoking.

CAUTION: If you have lung cancer, *do not* perform the Lion's Breath. The sudden increase in blood pressure as you sharply exhale can increase internal bleeding in the lungs.

MEDITATION AND GUIDED RELAXATION

In the West, most of us are busy spending the physical "bank account" of energy we inherit from our parents. We do not have a cultural tradition of restoring and even building this bank account.

Most Asian cultures have a long tradition of daily practices that restore physical, mental, emotional and spiritual health. Relaxation, contemplation, prayer, gentle physical exercise (e.g. qigong and yoga) and meditation all add "deposits" of energy in our life bank account.

The simplest form of meditation, known in both Eastern and Western cultures, is "replacing many minds with one mind." In Christian monasteries, for example, monks and nuns focus on a Bible verse or prayer. This singular focus replaces the usual ping-pong activity of the mind. The constantly shifting thoughts or "many minds" are replaced with the "single mind"—in this case, a Bible verse or prayer.

Another simple, effective focus is the breath. Take a moment now to observe breath moving through your nostrils. Can you sense the very edge of the nostril where breath first enters the body? Do you feel breath as it moves through the trachea and into the lungs? Watch the rise and fall of the belly. The aim is simply to observe, *not* to change the breath.

You can also add counting, to give your mind an additional point of focus. Observe the rise and fall of the chest. One. Air moving in the nostrils and out. Two. Belly expanding and relaxing. Three. Count up to 10 and then start over again.

You may also choose a particular word or phrase to repeat at the end of each exhalation. Choose a word or phrase that has meaning for you, that uplifts and supports your spirit as well as your body.

Walking meditation

You can bring the same mindful observation to walking. You may choose to walk in a quiet park, the back yard or your living room. If you are in a smaller area, make sure you have enough room to turn easily.

Begin walking with your arms swinging in a relaxed rhythm at your sides. Allow the eyes to focus softly in the distance, so that you are not rigidly focused on any one object. Keep the spine erect but not rigid.

Notice the sensation as your heel touches the ground and the muscle contractions as your toe pushes the foot behind you. Observe the sensations of muscles contracting and relaxing as you move forward.

As your attention moves deeper into your body, your steps likely will slow. Allow this to happen naturally. Remember that the purpose is to observe your walking, not to control it.

For more instruction and inspiration, refer to Thich Nhat Hanh's *Walking Meditation DVD/CD/Book Set* (Sounds True, Inc., 1996) or Sylvia Boorstein PhD's book *Don't Just Do Something: Sit There* (HarperOne, 1996).

GUIDED RELAXATION

You can find a myriad of recordings that guide you into a deeply relaxed state. You can visit my Web site at *www.drjudithboice.com/relaxation* for a guided relaxation recording. This is a wonderful practice before going to sleep or any time during the day when you need a "power nap."

Another wonderful tool, "Four-Route Relaxation," comes from qigong tradition (see below). This particular lying-down relaxation exercise has been practiced in China for 4-to-5,000 thousand years. Even terminally ill patients can practice this very effective form of rejuvenation.
http://drjudithboice.3dcartstores.com/Relaxation-CD_p_78.html

QIGONG

"Qi" (pronounced "tchee") means "life force" or "vitality"; *gong* means "skill" or "practice." Qigong is the skill or practice of increasing energy and vitality in the body.

I'm passionate about teaching my patients qigong because this practice allows them to build health between appointments. Instead of passively waiting for the next treatment or dose of supplements, they can actively rebuild their vitality on a daily basis.

From Chinese medical perspective, we inherit a store of *jing*, our prenatal essence or vitality that is stored in the kidneys. In addition to *jing*, the kidneys store *yin* and *yang*. *Yin* is the nourishing, cooling, fluid aspects of the body. *Yang* is all the heating and activating properties in the body. Together, *yin* and *yang* create a supportive unity, with one feeding the other, to each other's benefit.

Asian medicine and culture have a long history of cultivating and protecting *qi*, *jing*, *yin* and *yang*. Many Asian people engage in daily practices that build vitality and place "deposits" in their energy bank account, in the kidneys.

In contrast, most Westerners are busy spending the bank account, with no thought of replenishing it.

Qigong increases the vibratory rate of the body, so that disease can no longer inhabit the body. Think of running 1,000 volts of electricity through an appliance designed for 120 volts. The appliance would burn up and be destroyed.

Imagine that cancer and other diseases are geared for 120-volt, low vitality or low "electricity" states. If the "current" in the body begins to surge at 500 or 1,000 volts, the cancer can no longer survive.

Qigong rejuvenates every system, organ and gland in the body. We know from studies in China, the United States and other countries that qigong can address a wide variety of conditions and diseases:

- Cancer patients regularly practicing qigong better tolerated the side effects of chemotherapy and radiation treatments.
- Asthma patients missed fewer days of work and reported fewer symptoms with regular qigong practice.
- Multiple sclerosis patients who regularly practiced qigong had improved overall function.
- Qigong can help lower blood pressure; calm the nervous system; reduce or eliminate chronic pain; improve digestive function; and normalize immune function.

If you are interested in qigong, PLEASE learn from a qualified teacher. Qigong is transmitted as a living tradition. If you try to learn from a book or recording, you run the risk of creating what is called "deviation." This "deviation," or inappropriate flow of *qi*, is caused by incorrectly practicing qigong.

As an example, one of the students in a qigong teacher training suddenly developed ankle pain. She discussed the situation with her teacher, and they could not find any cause for the pain (e.g., hairline fracture of the ankle, sprain, etc.) An X-ray revealed no problem in the ankle.

Finally, the qigong instructor observed the student doing a particular qigong routine, a liver clearing form that moves tremendous energy down the leg and out the big toe. The teacher discovered that instead of slightly elevating her foot on a rock or tree root, the student had her foot flat on the ground. In this position, the energy could not move out the big toe; instead, it was accumulating in the ankle and causing great pain.

From Chinese medical perspective, lack of free flow causes pain. They envision these flows of energy through the body as rivers that are called meridians or channels. If the river is dammed or has run dry, the body experiences pain. In this case, the student had created a dam by placing her foot flat on the ground. Slightly elevating the foot on a rock or tree root opened the channel, allowing *qi* to flow freely. As soon as the student corrected her form by placing her foot on a tree root during the exercise, her ankle pain resolved.

This is one example of "deviation." This student's story illustrates the importance of working with a qualified teacher when you learn qigong. If she had been learning from a book, she would not have had someone to correct her form. At the very least, her incorrect practice would have caused ongoing pain; at worst, the incorrect practice might have caused more serious injury. Either way, the student likely would have abandoned qigong practice, claiming it had caused her pain. In truth, her *incorrect practice* of qigong is what caused the pain.

If you are interested in learning qigong, find a qualified teacher to learn from. Ask him about his training, where he studied and what form of qigong he teaches. If possible, ask the instructor to talk with her longtime students. Visit a class; participate in the form; and observe how your body responds.

Once you choose to study qigong, stay with a particular form for at least a year before moving on to learn additional forms. This first year is crucial in teaching the body to move *qi* in healthy ways. Trying to learn several new forms at once will create energetic "indigestion" in the body. Imagine first learning to dance and taking jazz, ballet, tap and modern dance all at once! Learning any one of the dance forms would create a solid foundation for learning others—at a later time.

In the West, some students collect qigong forms like baseball cards—"Oh, how many forms do *you* know?" In truth, a student could pursue one form for a lifetime while continuing to move deeper and deeper into its healing gifts. Depth of practice is much more important than the number of forms you know.

If you are interested in more information and a schedule of classes, please visit my Web site: *http://www.drjudithboice.com/qigong.html.*

INDIGENOUS MEDICINE

Years ago an editor called me shortly after my return from six months of living and traveling with traditional Aboriginal people in Australia.

"We're compiling a book of short health tips—you know, things that would help people improve their health. I know you just returned from living with Aboriginal people. Do you have any tips that you could submit?"

I was stymied about how to answer this editor's query. I truly wanted to help her with the book, but I could not fathom how to compress the profound complexity of Aboriginal culture into sound-bite "tips" for creating health. The editor wanted me to compress a rich, complex cuisine into denatured fast food.

Living with Aboriginal people, I came to understand that "health" rested upon ancient principles of right relationship with spirit, self, other humans and the Earth. How could I explain to the editor that the root of Aboriginal health was a profound connection with place, one that spanned over 40,000 years of interaction? How could I compress the intimate knowledge of desert plants, as well as how to find and harvest them, into a two-sentence sound bite? That relationship included not only an understanding of the plant as food and medicine, but also a "dream-time" story that taught a sense of place, morality and history, all at the same time.

I could have made some cryptic comments such as, "Get up every morning to watch the sunrise," which would have pointed to the richness and complexity of the Aboriginal culture. Having spent several weeks in Australia's Western Desert, at least 1,000 kilometers from the nearest paved road, I understood the importance of watching the sunrise. Just as Inuit people have many words for snow, the Martujarra people of the Western Desert have several words for the return of the light. In the West, we have the words "dawn" and "sunrise"; but we don't have names for the many subtle stages of light returning to the world.

After spending many weeks literally sleeping in the dirt in a land where temperatures dropped to freezing, the return of the light and, thus, heat in the arid desert was truly a phenomenon to observe and celebrate. The first glimmer of light at the horizon had a name, as did light strengthening to the point of outlining a bush or tree in the darkness. I considered myself to be an aware observer of the Earth, but the Martujarra had mastered levels of observation far beyond my relatively novice abilities.

Indigenous medicine refers to the healing methods of "primary people"— those who have had an unbroken relationship with the land and their culture over many millennia. This deep relationship with the land has spawned systems of healing that rely on principles foreign to conventional medicine.

The way someone gathers a plant, for example, has a profound impact on that plant's healing properties. Absent-mindedly ripping a plant from the ground and tossing it in a shed to dry produces an herb with different healing properties than one gathered with offerings and respect and then prepared with loving intention. Western medical researchers are beginning to understand that these respectful, even reverent ways of interacting with plants produce radically different results than we see with commercially prepared herbs.

Indigenous medicine draws its strength from people's relationship with the Earth *right where they live*. Instead of searching for exotic cures in other lands, they rely on the elements, plants and animals in their own back yard. They are not wooed by the hype about "ancient secrets" from some other culture; they are already aware of the miracles in their *own* region.

Medicine as right relationship

Indigenous medicine also focuses on more than the physical body, the plants and elements that surround us. The root of all indigenous medicines is right relationship with all aspects of creation. If I am taking the perfect herbs for my illness but still harbor fear, resentment, anger, or depression, the herbs cannot completely heal my whole being. Indigenous medicine addresses the physical body within the context of someone's entire life.

David Winston, a gifted Cherokee teacher, describes what his people call "ghost sickness." When people are completely disconnected from themselves and their community, they are diagnosed with this illness. The primary "cure" for "ghost sickness" is not herbs or foods; instead, the medicine person works with these displaced persons to reorient them to their soul. The "medicine" might involve working with the aged, the sick or the poor in the community. Ceremony would be an important part of realigning them to relationship with the self and with their community. These spiritual realignments are more important than chiropractic spinal adjustments or super-foods or the current "designer" herbal craze.

For native people, "medicine" is a way of life, not a pill or supplement. Although native healers do work with herbs and elements, the root of their healing comes from a profound connection with the land and with spirit. Without these relationships with earth and spirit, even the most perfect herbal remedy would be impotent in its effects. Moving and working *with* earth and spirit, miracles are possible and even commonplace.

As Master Lin Yun of Black Hat Sect Feng Shui tradition emphasized, *focusing intention with action produces 120-percent effect.* Combining right relationships with self, family, community and spirit with your healing intention can exponentially increase the effectiveness of your "cures."

CHAPTER 3

Treasures in the Green Medicine Chest

Use this chapter as a quick reference when you need to choose a remedy. Bookmark this section so you can return to it often.

The Green Medicine Chest includes:

- Herbs
- Homeopathics
- Essential oils
- Flower essences
- Castor oil and wool flannel
- Sea salt (neti pot and salt glow)
- Washcloths, towels
- Vegetable fiber brush (for skin brushing)

HOMEOPATHIC REMEDIES

These homeopathic descriptions paint a picture of the acute conditions that would benefit from taking the remedy. You do NOT have to have every single symptom for the remedy to be a good fit.

I might have a left-sided sore throat, for example, that improves after taking a dose of homeopathic Lachesis. I would not necessarily have other symptoms associated with Lachesis, e.g., I might not be restless, suspicious, chilly or talkative (loquacious).

The most characteristic guiding signs and symptoms for each remedy are in *italics*.

Aconitum napellus: Colds that begin after exposure to cold, dry winds. *Sudden onset* (within a few hours of exposure). Fever, intense thirst, *restlessness and anxiety*. Patient thinks s/he will die. Trembling. No sweating. Sphere of influence is the nervous system.

Allium cepa: allergic or cold symptoms with watery, teary eyes. Eyes excoriated, burning, sensitive to light (allergies). Bland, watery discharge from eyes, *excoriating discharge from nose* (influenza). Copious, acrid, watery discharges. Burning sensation of eyelids, nostrils, lips. (Think of how you feel when you are cutting onions). Worse indoors, in a warm room, in the evening. Better outdoors, or in a cold room.

Antimonium tartaricum: Cough with coarse rattling in the chest or larynx. Wet-sounding cough but scanty expectoration. Overwhelming sleepiness during cough or bronchitis. Weakened state; end-stage disease. Feeble pulse. Bronchitis in infants; also elderly patients, especially in winter months. Chicken pox. Cyanosis with respiratory conditions (lack of oxygen leads to blue lips, face, fingernail beds, etc.).

Apis mellifica: *Swollen, red, irritated skin or mucous membrane tissue* (e.g., back of the throat). Remember how a bee sting feels: *burning, itching, rapid swelling*. Better with cold applications. Excellent for *insect bites, sunburn, hives*. Severely swollen, sore throats. Worse with heat and touch. Better in the open air.

Arnica montana: *Classic for soft tissue injuries, bruising, trauma. Concussion, head injury. Hemorrhage.* Take before and after dental work. Take a dose as soon as possible after an injury, e.g., a sprained ankle, bumped or bruised limb, auto accident and/or head injury. Sphere of influence is vascular system. With onset of *shock, the head is hot and the rest of the body weak.* The patient often will *deny being hurt* and say that he does not need help. She may feel as if she is going to die. Worse with motion, touch, cold and cold damp. Better lying down, head low.

Arsenicum album: Effects the *mucous membranes* (lining of digestive tract, lungs). *Intense burning pains.* Can't stand the sight or smell of food. *Food poisoning, with vomiting and diarrhea.* "Fire hydrant stools." Restlessness, weakness, pain, headaches. *Intense aversion to sunlight (photophobia). Thirsty; wants frequent sips of warm water. Chilly. Worse after midnight. Anxious, restless, fearful. Headache.*

Belladonna: Sudden, violent onset of illness characterized by fever and severe pain. Key symptoms are *intense heat, redness, throbbing and swelling.* Face is red, hot, dry; the skin seems to radiate heat. The rest of body is sweating. *No thirst,* despite mouth being dry. Head is hot; limbs are cold. Eyes are glassy, staring; pupils are dilated. Oversensitive to noise and light. Appears dull, dazed. May become *angry* and violent. May have hallucinations. Better lying down, lying on abdomen. *Colds, fevers, headaches.*

Borax: Travel sickness, especially air travel with air pockets. *Dread of downward motion. Very sensitive to noise and pain.* Worse from salt and spicy food, sudden noises, cold, wet, least uncovering. May help resolve canker sores (mouth is hot and dry, red mucus, will bleed if touched).

Bryonia alba: Flu-like illnesses. Everything is *worse with motion. Better lying on painful part* (strange, rare and peculiar symptom). *Intense thirst. Patient drinks lots of water.* Fatigue. Irritable, angry; wants to be left alone. Joint pains worse with motion. Dryness also is characteristic, e.g., dry mouth, eyes, throat. Constipation. Better with rest, heat on inflamed part, cool room.

Calcarea carbonica (Calc carb): Classic children's remedy. Primary sphere of influence is calcium-rich structures (bone, teeth). *Cradle cap. Stubborn,* slow moving. *Teeth slow to erupt.* Late beginning to walk. Adults: *constipation with no urge for stool. Back weakness and low back pain. Arthritis,* worse cold and damp; worse exertion (opposite Rhus tox).

Cantharis: Keynotes are *burning pains. Burns and scalds,* with a feeling of painful rawness that is better with cold applications. *Cutting, smarting, burning pains,* e.g., after a burn or bladder infection. *Second-degree burn with blister formation.*

Chamomilla: *Nerve pain,* especially associated with teething and earaches. Pain is so acute the patient is *screaming.* Thirsty, restless. The child is irritable and wants to be held, but when she is picked up, she *screams and arches back.* Child doesn't know what he wants. *One cheek is red; the other is pale.* Better: being carried, sweating, cold applications. Worse: anger, night, dentition, wind, open air. *If the child is calm, Chamomilla is the wrong remedy.*

Cinchona officinalis: *Debility after excessive loss of fluids,* e.g., blood, saliva, breast milk (nursing), semen, vaginal discharge and/or diarrhea. *Late-stage remedy.* Hemorrhage with faintness, loss of sight and ringing in the ears. *Periodicity – every other day. Nervous. Sensitive to drafts, slightest touch.* Chronic gout. Post-operative gas pains; no relief from passing it. *Better: hard pressure on painful part;* open air; warmth. *Worse: slightest touch, draft of air, every other day, after eating.*

Cocculus indicus: Travel sickness (sea and car sickness) associated with nausea, dizziness. *Sense of emptiness in head; hollow feeling.* Cannot lie on back part of head. Averse to food. Sensitive to cold. Insomnia due to stress.

Colocynthis: Cramping, *abdominal pain that is better bending double.* Menstrual or colicky pains. Small amount of food or drink causes violent diarrhea. *Jelly-like stools. Pains are better with hard pressure.*

Dulcamara: Aggravation from cold damp weather (conjunctivitis, diarrhea, bladder infection, low back pain). Aggravated from change in weather, from catching cold. Headache from suppressed sinusitis. Urging for urination when chilled. Rheumatism. Hayfever, end of summer or in fall.

Drosera rotundifolia: *Violent cough*, sometimes so severe the patient *cannot catch his breath and begins to turn blue.* Cough is *worse after midnight.* Cough associated with *pertussis (whooping cough).* The cough is severe enough to cause a nosebleed. Cough is worse lying down, worse in the warmth of bed. Drosera also addresses *muscle cramping,* particularly hand cramps and shoulder twitches.

Eupatorium perfoliatum: Tremendous aching, as if the bones were broken. Back pain, excruciating. Colds, flu, fever with deep, aching bone pain. Chilly, with tremendous thirst for cold drinks.

Euphrasia officinalis: Hay fever symptoms. Eye inflammation and tearing. *Bland discharge from nose. Acrid discharge/tearing from eyes* (opposite of Allium cepa). *Eyes constantly water.* Worse: sunlight, wind, being indoors. Better: open air, winking, wiping eyes, lying down.

Ferrum Phosphoricum (Ferrum phos): *Early stages of febrile illness,* e.g., colds and the flu. Bleeding, e.g., coughing blood streaked sputum; nosebleeds in children. *High fever with few symptoms.*

Gelsemium sempervirens: For slow onset colds, often occurring in mild or warm weather. The remedy is often prescribed for *colds during warm winters.* Patient is *dull, dizzy, droopy, drowsy ("the four D's").* No thirst. Feels as if she has a band around her head. Muscle weakness, dropping things, uncoordinated. The common name for the remedy is Swamp Jasmine: Think of how you would feel in a hot, muggy, humid swamp in August. Helpful for *stagefright, test anxiety* (patient is worse with dread, emotions, surprise). With *shock,* patient is drowsy, droopy, dull. They may be confused, dazed and apathetic. Pupils may be dilated, with drooping eyelids. Patient wants to sleep. May be indicated for heat stroke.

Hepar sulphuris calcareum (Hepar sulph): Colds that begin after exposure to north and northeast wind (this was described by a homeopath on the East Coast, so think of a Nor'easter storm): cold, dry, windy weather. *Sticking pain in throat. Sharp, stitching pain in ear. Extreme sensitivity to pain.* Irritable, nasty. *Cannot tolerate exposure to cold or wind.* Much perspiration. Excellent remedy for *otitis media* (ear infection) with discharge. *Helps resolve or bring boils to a head.*

Hypericum perforatum: Damage to nerves, e.g., slamming a finger in a car door. Crush injuries, lacerations of fingers, fingertips. Painful wounds. Nerve pain. Worse: touch, jarring, cold. First-degree sunburn. Sciatica.

Ignatia amara: A remedy for *grief,* with sensation of a *lump in the throat* and much *sighing. Contradictory symptoms,* e.g., throat pain is worse swallowing water but better swallowing solids. *Worse: smoking or smelling tobacco. Oversensitive, nervous. Hysterical crying.*

Ipecacuanha (Ipecac): *Nausea, vomiting, dry heaves.* Violent, persistent nausea. Nerve to stomach becomes irritated and vomiting continues despite empty stomach. *Dry, nagging cough.* Patient coughs so hard and so long that she vomits or has dry heaves. Asthma with a violent cough; coughs with every breath.

Kali bichromicum: *Cough with thick, stringy mucous,* difficult to expectorate. Hoarse. Worse in the evening. Patient is *chilly* and thirsty.

Lachesis mutus: *Left-sided complaints,* e.g., left-sided sore throat, or sore throat that travels left → right. Worse from touch; *cannot tolerate anything around the neck. Worse touch in general.* Sleeps into aggravation (is worse on waking). *Left-sided sciatica,* worse at night and cold air. *Loquacious.* Restless, suspicious, chilly.

Ledum palustre: *Puncture wounds,* e.g., injury by a sharp object or insect bite. *Bruising with feeling of coldness; blueness* of affected part. Affected part is cold, *but better cold applications* (strange, rare and peculiar symptom). Thirsty. *Chilly.*

Lycopodium clavatum: *Digestive complaints,* intestinal gas, bloating. *Worse from 4-8 p.m. Right-sided complaints.* Sore throats that are worse on right side or travel right → left. Burning pain between scapulae; pain goes right → left. Right-sided sciatica. *Hard, difficult, incomplete stool* ("bashful stool"). Hates tight clothing around the waist.

Magnesia Phosphorica (Mag phos): *Muscle cramping,* e.g., leg cramps, menstrual cramps. *Better with warm application.*

Mercurius vivus: Inflammation of mucous membranes and skin with pus formation; raw, open areas. Tonsillitis, sore throat with desire to swallow. *Excessive salivation. Breath is foul-smelling. Sensitive to temperature changes (hot/cold,* like the mercury in a thermometer). Worse at night. Trembling, jerking of limbs, tongue. Affected tissues slow to heal. Metallic taste in the mouth. *Agitated, restless, rapid talking. Mind is dull and sluggish.*

Natrum muriaticum (Nat mur): Grief, often silent. Holds feelings in. Sad, yet unable to cry. Does not want to be consoled. Headache, especially from close work (e.g., reading). Migraine headache. Headache "like hammers beating the head." Headache from grief. Better lying in a dark, quiet room; better cold applications. Hayfever. Asthma, worse in the evenings, 7-to-9 p.m. Herpetic eruptions (cold sores), especially after sun exposure. In general, dislikes sun exposure.

Nux vomica: Indigestion or uneasiness following overeating and/or excessive drinking. "Hangover." Impatient, irritable. Headache. Wants to be left alone. Sensitive to noise, light, odors, pressure of clothing. Angry. Chilly. With cold or flu, stuffed up at night, more fluent nasal discharge during the day. Body is burning hot but cannot move or uncover without feeling a chill or refuses being covered even though chilled with uncovering. Worse drinking coffee or taking stimulants.

Oscillococcinum: *For the very onset of cold/flu symptoms (first 24 hours).* Anxious, pale, shivering; fixed, obsessive ideas.

Phosphorus: Bleeding. Red, arterial blood flow. Nosebleeds. May be used after surgery to decrease risk of hemorrhage. Desires cold drinks but vomits them as soon as they warm in the stomach. Better eating, sleeping. Desires company. Worse talking—may have painless laryngitis. Colds that quickly go to the lungs. Cough so painful patient tries to suppress it. Blood-streaked sputum.

Podophyllum peltatum: *Diarrhea.* Colicky pains and sour vomiting. Watery stools. *Thirst for large quantities of cold water.* Diarrhea in hot weather after eating acid fruits. *Painless, watery diarrhea.*

Pulsatilla: the common name is "wind flower" because it moves with every breath of wind. Keynote is *changeable symptoms,* e.g., joint pains that move around the body. "Ripe" colds with green/yellow, thick discharge. Cough is looser in the morning, drier as the day goes on. Infection of the tear duct, or blocked tear duct, in infants and newborns. *Weepy. Thirstless, with dry mouth. Desires open air. Worse in a warm room.* Timid, mild.

Rhus toxicodendron: Joint pains that are better *with movement. Restless,* can't find a comfortable position. *Chilly. Thirsty.* Worse after exposure to cold and wet. Colds that begin after exposure to cold and wet. Red tip of tongue. *Itching, burning, stinging of skin. Vesicular eruptions. Sensation as if flesh has been torn from the bone.* Better from scalding hot water, showers. Chilly.

Ruta graveolens: Damage to *ligaments and periosteal tissue* (area around bone). *Pain comes in waves.* Pain deep in the bones. Eyestrain from reading small print or close-up work, especially if followed by a headache. Worse from cold, wet weather; overexertion; damp; wind. Follows Arnica well for sprains.

Sepia: Loss of tissue integrity, e.g., prolapsed uterus, hemorrhoids, varicose veins. Symptoms generally worse with any hormonal fluctuation, e.g., before and during menstruation; PMS; pregnancy; menopause; frequent sex. Mother is angry and yells at the children from least disturbance; worst while cooking dinner. Made from octopus ink; think of the purpose of the ink—to conceal and be left alone.

Silicea: Late stage, chronic colds. Recurring sore throats and tonsillitis. Hard, swollen cervical glands. Acute ear infections, as well as ear infections that are very slow to resolve. Infection of the tear duct, or blocked tear duct, in infants and newborns. Defects of bone, spine, nails and hair, from poor mineral absorption. Constipation with no urging; bashful stool (almost comes out, then recedes again). Constipation in children. Helps to discharge splinters, foreign substances from the body.

Spongia tosta: *Dry, hacking cough.* Imagine inhaling dried sponge and what that would feel like. Larynx dry, constricted, burning. *Barking, croupy cough.* Croup worse during inspiration. Anxiety. Better leaning forward. Better eating a little. One of three classic croup remedies: Aconite, Spongia, Hepar sulph. The three remedies are used in the order listed: Aconite for onset of symptoms, Spongia for the mid-illness symptoms (dry, hacking cough) and Hepar sulph for the last stage of croup.

Sulphur: Important remedy for skin eruptions. Dry skin, *itching;* roughness. *Voluptuous itching.* Will scratch until skin bleeds. Thirsty. *Worse warmth –* warm room, warm bed. Sleeps with window open. Feet so hot the patient uncovers them in bed. *Burning discharges and pains. Skin and face reddened.* Offensive discharges, odors. *Worse from bathing.* Impatient, hurried, quick-tempered, opinionated. Late stages of viral infections.

Symphytum officinale: "Arnica of the eye," specific for *bruising around the eye. Orbital fractures. Give the remedy on the way to the Emergency Room.* Pain associated with bruising and fracture. Cartilage or bone injuries. Periosteal (outer layer of bone) injuries (Ruta as well). *Fractures that fail to heal.*

BOTANICALS

Arnica Oil (*Arnica montana*): For bruising and soft tissue injury. Apply only on unbroken skin. Best applied immediately after injury. Can help prevent bruising and reduce swelling. CAUTION: Never take Arnica HERB internally. *Homeopathic* arnica (see above) is *safe* for internal use.

Aloe (*Aloe barbadensis*): The inner gel of the aloe plant is soothing, anti-inflammatory and anti-pruritic (reduces itching). The gel speeds tissue healing, e.g., for gastric ulcers, bedsores and diabetic skin ulcers. The outer "skin" of the aloe plant contains a bitter latex that acts as a "cathartic," dramatically clearing the bowels. This outer skin is helpful for short-term use, to address severe constipation. Long-term use, though, will deplete electrolytes and further weaken the muscles in the bowel. Constitutional hydrotherapy (see Hydrotherapy in Chapter 2) offers a more permanent "cure" for constipation.

Bentonite clay: A drawing agent, to remove pus and inflammation from an affected area such as an infected cut or poison ivy/oak. Can be taken internally for diarrhea and mild food poisoning.

Bilberry (*Vaccinium myrtilis*) The berries and leaves improve circulation and strengthen blood vessel walls, making bilberry a wonderful ally for retinopathy, cataracts, macular degeneration and night blindness. Bilberry also improves microcirculation in other parts of the body and minimizes bruising.

Bitter melon fruit (*Momardica charantia*) Bitter melon stabilizes blood sugar levels and suppresses the usual neural response to sweet taste. Commonly eaten in India and Southeast Asia, bitter melon also inhibits retroviruses (HIV, herpes) and is cytotoxic (kills cancer cells, e.g., leukemia and certain types of breast cancer).

Blue vervain (*Verbena hostata*) Blue vervain is a diaphoretic (causes sweating) and is used to treat fevers and colds as well as clear bronchial congestion.

Black cohosh (*Cimicifuga racemosa*) High in calcium, black cohosh relieves smooth muscle cramps, e.g., menstrual pain. Black cohosh also relieves muscle spasms and joint pain. For menopause, black cohosh seems to have some phytoestrogen effect (not fully confirmed in recent studies). In addition, black cohosh suppresses leutenizing hormone surges, which are associated with hot flashes in menopause. Black cohosh relaxes the smooth muscle in blood vessels, which improves blood circulation in the extremities.

Buckthorn bark (*Cascara sagrada*): Stimulates peristalsis. Some people experience intestinal cramping with cascara. With long-term use, cascara can have the same side effects as chemical laxatives, so short-term usage (2 weeks maximum) is best during the bowel retraining program.

Calendula succus (*Calendula officinalis*): "Succus" means plant juice. Tinctures are about 70% alcohol and approximately 30% plant extract. Succus preparations are about 70% plant extract with about 30% alcohol—they contain much more of the active constituents of the plant. Calendula is an excellent antimicrobial that also has vulnerary (soothing, healing) properties. Apply after washing the wound. Calendula can replace washing a clean wound in an emergency situation. Calendula succus is more effective at halting bacterial growth than iodine solutions or rubbing alcohol.

Calendula and comfrey salve: Calendula has antimicrobial and vulnerary properties. Comfrey (*Symphytum officinale*) stimulates cell division and thus speeds wound healing. Best applied to clean cuts only or ones that have formed a scab, not to puncture wounds (may cause the skin to heal over a dirty wound, creating an anaerobic environment perfect for the growth of anaerobic bacteria).

Catnip (*Nepeta cataria*) A calming nervine, catnip also increases sweating without raising internal body temperature, making this a wonderful herb for feverish children. Catnip also soothes restlessness, nervous headaches, insomnia and menstrual cramping. CAUTION: Contraindicated during pregnancy because of its emmenagogue effect (brings on menstruation).

Chamomile (*Matricaria rescutita*) High in calcium, chamomile gently soothes the nervous system and helps prepare for sleep. Chamomile reduces spasms and inflammation, relieves pain, calms the stomach and improves digestive function. In addition, chamomile has anti-bacterial and anti-fungal activity.

Comfrey (*Symphytum officinale*) Comfrey contains allantoin, a constituent that speeds cell division and, therefore, tissue healing. Comfrey also has anti-inflammatory effect, easing bone and tendon inflammation. Comfrey is mucilaginous, soothing both the respiratory and digestive tracts. Although historically used internally to reduce inflammation and speed tissue healing, current research suggests extremely large amounts of pyrrolizidine alkaloid in comfrey can occlude veins and trigger carcinogenic (cancer) activity. CAUTION: Take internally only under the guidance of a trained herbalist. Do not use if pregnant or nursing.

Dandelion root and leaf (*Taraxacum officinalis*) Dandelion leaf has a strong diuretic effect, increasing urination and decreasing fluid retention. Collect the greens early in the spring for a wonderful spring salad. Dandelion root is a mild laxative that triggers bile secretion from the liver. Dandelion *slowly* stimulates liver function, so you will need to use the herb over time. Collect dandelion roots in the autumn, when they contain maximum nutrients.

Echinacea (*Echinacea angustifolia OR purpurea*) Echinacea does *not* directly "attack" bacteria; instead, it stimulates immune activity by increasing white blood cell production. Some studies suggest Echinacea loses its efficacy after two to three weeks of continuous use; most studies show Echinacea is very effective with long-term use. For maximum effect, consider alternating immune-boosting herbs every two to three weeks to ensure their efficacy.

Elderberry (*Sambucus pubens*) Elder *berries* are used to treat colds, the flu, joint pain and nerve pain. The *flowers*, more commonly used in botanical medicine, help to expel mucous, increase sweating and calm the nervous system. Elder flowers can be used for chronic sinus irritation, night sweats, spasmodic coughs and skin eruptions. CAUTION: Unripe elder berries can cause nausea, vomiting, dizziness, fast heart rate and convulsions. Use only fully ripened berries.

Ginger (*Zingiber officinalis*) Ginger warms the body, increasing sweating and improving digestion. Dried ginger has more "heating" effect than the fresh root. Ginger decreases platelet aggregation, meaning it slows blood clotting time (use with caution if taking Coumadin or other anti-coagulants). Ginger *tincture* is very effective for addressing post-chemotherapy nausea, but ginger *tea* has little effect. Ginger also has anti-inflammatory properties, making it a wonderful ally for joint and muscle pain. Fresh ginger juice can be used topically to treat first- and second-degree burns.

Ginseng: Korean, Chinese (*Panax ginseng*) and American (*Panax quinque-folius*) Ginseng is an adaptogen herb, meaning it helps the body better adapt to stress levels. Ginseng supports the nervous and hormonal systems; stabilizes blood sugar; reduces LDL and increases HDL cholesterol; improves metabolic activity in the brain; and minimizes cell damage and hastens recovery from radiation exposure. In Chinese medicine, ginseng is considered a *qi* tonic, meaning it helps to rebuild vitality in the body. American ginseng tonifies both *qi* and *yin*, meaning it also enhances the nourishing, moistening and cooling aspects of the body. Chinese ginseng is considered more heating, while Korean is the "hottest" of the three ginsengs. Usually Asian people do not take ginseng regularly before they are 60 years old; otherwise, they have already "boosted" their body with this potent tonic and have nothing left to further enhance their vitality. In essence, they have "shot their wad" too early.

Goldenseal (*Hydrastis canadensis*) Goldenseal is a *mucous membrane* **tonic**, affecting the entire digestive and respiratory tracts. Goldenseal can be used for upper respiratory infections as well as digestive disturbances, e.g., stomach pains and gas after eating.

Goldenthread (*Coptis chinensis*) A century ago, herbalists began to substitute Goldenseal (*Hydrastis canadensis*) for Goldenthread because the roots of Goldenthread were being over-harvested. Ironically, herbalists now recommend Goldenthread as a substitute for increasingly rare Goldenseal. Both of these bitter roots are high in berberine, a compound known to kill bacteria, viruses and fungi. Goldenthread also stimulates digestive function (e.g., saliva and stomach acid secretion), reduces inflammation and lowers high blood cholesterol levels. Goldenthread also calms the nervous system and relieves pain, helping to soothe abdominal cramps, muscle aches, irritability and insomnia.

Gymnema sylvestra Grown in India, this plant stabilizes blood sugar levels and reduces sweet taste on the tongue, thereby reducing sugar cravings. This herb is used to treat diabetes and pre-diabetes, i.e., difficulty regulating blood sugar levels.

Hawthorne berry (*Crataegus species*) Most herbalists combine hawthorne berries and flowers. Hawthorne increases the strength and efficiency of heart contractions and has mild diuretic effect. Meant for long-term use and not acute illnesses, hawthorne also increases blood flow in the heart and enhances connective tissue strength of blood and lymph vessels. Hawthorne improves overall cardiac function.

Hops (*Humulus lupulus*): Soothes irritable digestive tract and nervous system (indigestion and sleeplessness). Hops is very specific for soothing nervousness with muscle twitching. This muscle-relaxing property also makes hops a wonderful aide for menstrual cramping. For nursing mothers, drinking hops tea increases milk production, soothes both mother and baby and addresses colic in the infant.

Kava kava (*Piper methysticum*): This nervine herb calms the nervous system without sedating the mind. Kava relieves anxiety and stress, insomnia and muscle tension. Caution: Long-term, high-dose use of Kava can cause dry, pigmented, scaly skin, particularly on the palms of the hands, soles of the feet, back and shins. This condition, called "kavaism," is more common in the South Pacific where people drink Kava like North Americans drink coffee. The rash disappears when someone stops drinking Kava Kava tea.

Lemon balm (*Melissa officinalis*) Used as a topical gel or essential oil, lemon balm can avert a herpes outbreak if applied frequently during the prodrome (pre-outbreak) phase. Regular external applications of lemon balm after an outbreak will also speed the healing of herpes lesions by about 2.5 days. Taken internally, e.g., as a tea, dried herb, or tincture, lemon balm has a calming effect on the nervous system, soothing anxiety and conditions worsened by nervousness. Lemon balm addresses colds, migraines, depression, high blood pressure and insomnia, especially when high stress levels contribute to the illness. Lemon balm blocks the binding of TSH to thyroid membrane cells, making it an excellent remedy for the treatment of hyperthyroidism (*over*-active thyroid).

Licorice (*Glycerrhiza glabra*) Another of the adaptogen herbs, licorice stimulates immune function, enhances adrenal activity, soothes inflammation, protects the liver and has mild estrogenic activity. In Chinese medicine, licorice is called "the great peacemaker." Most Chinese formulae contain a small amount of licorice to help harmonize the activity of the other herbs. CAUTION: Because licorice increases the biological half-life of cortisol and aldosterone, it may contribute to increased fluid retention. If you suffer with hypertension, use only *de-glycerrhinated licorice* (DGL) and watch carefully for any side effects. Licorice is also contraindicated for heart failure, kidney disease and liver cirrhosis.

Motherwort (*Leonorus cardiaca*) Truly an ally for women's health, motherwort soothes menstrual cramps and premenstrual nerve tension and brings on delayed menstrual bleeding. In addition, motherwort relieves heart palpitations due to nervous tension and soothes the pain of cold sores and genital herpes. Use motherwort for several months for best results.

Mullein (*Verbascum thapsus*) Use the leaves and flowers of mullein to soothe coughs and bronchitis, asthma and hay fever. Soak the flowers in vegetable oil for a couple of weeks, then strain out the flowers to make an oil for soothing ear pain. CAUTION: Use mullein oil in the external ear canal only if the tympanic membrane (ear drum) is NOT ruptured.

Nettles (*Urtica urens*) Nettles are a wonderful ally for treating seasonal hay fever because they stabilize the mast cells that release histamine, thereby reducing inflammation and swelling. In addition, nettles act as a mild diuretic and help to rebuild the urinary tract. Nettles are best used long-term, over several months, to achieve these rejuvenating effects.

Oregon grape root (*Berberis aquafolium*) Like Goldenthread and Goldenseal, Oregon grape root contains berberines, compounds that stimulate bile secretion; kill bacteria, viruses and fungi; and stimulate the digestive tract. Oregon grape root will stimulate and support the digestive, respiratory and urinary systems.

Passion flower (*Passiflora incarnata*): This herb soothes muscle spasms, heart palpitations and nervousness. Passion flower helps support normal sleep, particularly when nervousness contributes to sleep disturbances.

Peppermint (*Mentha piperita*) Peppermint relieves spasms, increases bile secretion, calms the stomach, dissolves gallstones and increases sweating (diaphoretic). Used on the skin, peppermint relieves the pain and itching of bug bites and soothes muscle spasms. CAUTION: Peppermint relaxes the lower gastroesophageal sphincter, which can worsen hiatal hernia and gastroesophageal reflux (GERDS) symptoms. In addition, avoid using peppermint during acute gallstone episodes.

Red clover blossoms (*Trifolium pratens*) A mild phytoestrogen (weak plant-based estrogen), red clover addresses estrogen dominance conditions (e.g., PMS, uterine fibroids and fibrocystic breasts) as well as provides weak estrogen support for low-estrogen conditions (e.g., hot flashes). Red clover soothes swollen lymph nodes, particularly in the neck region. CAUTION: Red clover thins the blood and must be used with caution if taking a blood thinner.

Rhodiola (*Rhodiola rosea*) A potent adaptogen herb, Rhodiola improves physical and mental performance; addresses depression and anxiety; reduces fatigue; improves memory and concentration; and increases tolerance to cold and other extreme weather conditions.

Saint John's Wort (*Hypericum perforatum*) Used for centuries to address nerve and spinal cord injuries, St. John's Wort is best known today for treating depression, increasing serotonin and melatonin levels and possibly increasing light utilization. For depression, St. John's Wort must be taken for at least 2-to-6 weeks to evaluate its effectiveness. St. John's Wort also treats viral infections.

Saint John's Wort (*Hypericum perforatum*) Oil: Soothing and feeding to the nervous system, St. John's Wort oil can speed the healing of nerve injuries, bruises and muscular pain. Helps relieve the pain of **sunburn**. Applied frequently, hypericum oil acts as a sunblock. Can relieve or abort sciatica if applied at earliest signs of pain and discomfort.

Saw palmetto (*Serenoa repens*) Known primarily as a men's herb, Saw palmetto reduces the size of the prostate gland and tonifies the entire pelvic region. For women, Saw palmetto stimulates breast development, increases libido and addresses polycystic ovaries. For both men and women, Saw palmetto may benefit interstitial cystitis and chronic bladder infections.

Senna (*Cassia senna*) Senna addresses constipation by increasing peristalsis, the wave-like muscle contractions that move food and waste through the digestive tract. Senna speeds intestinal movement by *irritating* the digestive tract. If used long-term, Senna increases melanosis, a darkened pigment in the colon, which *might* increase risk of colon cancer. CAUTION: Do not use if you have a history of kidney damage or kidney inflammation. Over-use may cause vomiting, intestinal spasms and/or bloody diarrhea.

Siberian ginseng (*Eleuthorococcus senticosus*) This herb is another potent adaptogen herb. Although "ginseng" is in the name, this herb is a completely different genus from *Panax* ginseng. Siberian ginseng increases endurance, improves oxygenation of tissues, enhances concentration and increases overall resistance to disease.

Skullcap (*Scutellaria lateriflora*) – High in calcium, magnesium and potassium, this herb calms and nourishes the nervous system. Skullcap is beneficial for anxiety, restless sleep, nervous exhaustion and nervous system weakness after a long illness.

Slippery elm bark (*Ulmus fulva*) This mucilaginous inner bark of the slippery elm tree soothes the digestive and urinary tracts. Slippery elm bark reduces inflammation and acts as a mild diuretic. You can cook slippery elm bark powder by itself or with oatmeal to create a nutritious gruel. You can also suck on slippery elm bark lozenges to soothe the throat, stomach, intestines and/or urinary tract.

Valerian (*Valeriana officinalis*): Beloved by cats, this herb smells like dirty socks to me. Others love its pungent taste. Valerian relaxes skeletal muscle, particularly in the low back region, and relieves menstrual cramping. Too much valerian can have opposite effects, actually stimulating the nervous system rather than soothing it. CAUTION: Valerian can potentiate (increase) the action of barbiturates. AVOID combining valerian with any barbiturate medication.

Yarrow (*Achillea millefolium*) A tea made from infusing yarrow blossoms in *hot* water increases sweating, while infusing the herb in *cold* water increases the diuretic and gastric toning effects of yarrow. Because yarrow astringes tissues, it is an ally for hemorrhoids and excessive menstrual flow. Yarrow's botanical name reflects this ability to staunch blood flow: When an arrow pierced the god Achilles' heel, he used yarrow to stop the bleeding.

Yellow dock (*Rumex crispus*) The bitter roots of yellow dock stimulate bile secretion, improve bowel elimination and increase iron absorption. Also a good source of iron, yellow dock can be used to treat iron deficiency anemia. Yellow dock improves lymph flow and function. Use yellow dock for anemia, constipation, chronic skin conditions and liver congestion.

Chinese herbal formulae

Gan Mao Ling: This formula treats the very onset of colds, whether they are wind heat (sore throat, fever, sweating) or wind cold (chills, no sore throat, clear nasal discharge) in nature.

Pill Curing: This classic Chinese formula soothes nausea, vomiting, belching and acid stomach. You can take Pill Curing 30-to-60 minutes before traveling to allay motion sickness.

Xiao yao san: Translated "Free and Easy Wanderer," this formula enhances liver function and supports the production and free flow of blood in the body. From Chinese perspective, one of the liver's major roles is to smoothly circulate blood in the body. If blood flows smoothly, emotions also flow easily. When the liver is stressed and cannot circulate blood as smoothly, we are more prone to certain emotions: frustration, anger and/or depression. Physical symptoms may include menstrual cramping, PMS symptoms and/or sluggish digestion.

Yin qiao san: a Chinese patent medicine for "wind heat invasion." Symptoms include sore throat, feeling more feverish than chilled, slight headache and yellowish mucus discharge. Do not take the remedy if you feel more chills than fever and have no sore throat—the formula is *very* cooling. Yin qiao san is meant to cause sweating to help push out wind and heat. Make sure to avoid drafts and chills after taking the remedy.

Yunnan Pai Yao: is a Chinese herbal formula that was brought to the West from Vietnam, where U.S. soldiers witnessed its seemingly miraculous effects.

The powder can be taken internally or packed into wounds to stop bleeding. Each package includes one small red pill that is used only for severe hemorrhaging. The orange-powder capsules may be taken internally, one pill 3-to-4 times per day, to stop bleeding. Stop taking the medicine as soon as the bleeding stops.

ESSENTIAL OILS

Cypress (*Cupressus sempervirens*) Cypress fights bacteria, reduces spasms and calms the nervous system. Cypress is an even more effective astringent than witch hazel.

Eucalyptus globulus A powerful bronchodilator, this essential oil also has anti-viral, anti-fungal and anti-bacterial properties. Eucalyptus fights infection and thins mucous with coughs and bronchitis. Eucalyptus can also be used to treat Candida, sunburn and bladder infections. Diluted in a mister bottle with water, eucalyptus is an effective insect repellant.

Eucalyptus radiata Milder than *Eucalyptus globulus*, this species of Eucalyptus is appropriate for children and for skin applications.

Everlasting (*Helichrysum italicum*) Helichrysum is the "arnica" of the essential oil world. Applied immediately after an injury, Helichrysum can minimize or sometimes even avoid bruising and swelling. Apply on unbroken tissue. Helichrysum can be applied "neat," without diluting in a vegetable oil. Most helichrysum, however, is sold in diluted form because it is a very expensive essential oil. For old scars and stretch marks, apply a 20% dilution regularly over 2-to-3 months. Also reduces inflammation and swelling with insect stings.

Lavender (*Lavendula officinalis*) Lavender reduces inflammation, soothes burns and calms the nervous system. Lavender can be used to improve sleep, reduce pain, heal burns and other injuries and soothe migraine headaches. Lavender also has mild antiseptic properties and will speed tissue healing. Anti-venomous for insect and snake bites, lavender is also adaptogenic (helps the body better adapt to stress). Lavender also harmonizes the action of essential oils, making it a great addition to essential oil blends.

Peppermint (*Mentha piperita*): Peppermint has amphoteric action on the digestive tract, meaning it both soothes and stimulates the mucous membrane lining. One drop of peppermint essential oil in a cup of hot water will soothe an upset stomach. A drop rubbed into the temples may relieve a simple tension headache. One or two drops mixed with clay can soothe poison ivy/oak rash.

Peppermint helps relieve pain. Mixing 2-to-3 drops in vegetable oil and rubbing on the belly can soothe an upset stomach. CAUTION: Peppermint and other mints may antidote the actions of homeopathic remedies. Peppermint relaxes the cardiac sphincter of the stomach, so do NOT use peppermint if you have a hiatal hernia or gastroesophageal reflux (GERDS). Peppermint will worsen these conditions.

Tea Tree (*Melaleuca alternifolia*) This potent antiseptic oil is anti-fungal, anti-viral and anti-bacterial. Tea tree stimulates the immune system, specifically T-cell production. Tea tree is one of the few essential oils that can be applied "neat," without diluting in a vegetable oil. Six months after opening the bottle, however, the oil becomes more caustic and should be diluted in vegetable oil. You can use tea tree for athlete's foot, Candida, ringworm, toothache and pyorrhea. Add a drop of essential oil on your toothbrush for gum disease. Tea tree oil is the only essential oil that can be used vaginally, i.e., 2-to-3 drops on a tampon inserted once daily. Tea tree is also anti-venomous (i.e., treats insect, spider and snake bites).

Thyme (*Thymus vulgarus*) A strong anti-viral, thyme is an excellent choice for misting the house to prevent colds and the flu. You can also use thyme to treat warts, acne, nerve pain and joint pain. Thyme is an extremely potent essential oil and must be used with care. Always dilute this oil in a carrier vegetable oil and avoid using with children, unless you use thyme linalol, a gentler chemo-type of thyme essential oil.

FLOWER ESSENCES

- Baby Blue Eyes: no longer trusting the goodness in the world; cynicism.
- Bleeding Heart: for a broken heart, from loss of someone held very dear. Emotional codependence.
- Borage: discouragement, despair, heavy-heartedness. Lack of confidence facing difficulties.
- California Wild Rose: not accepting difficulty or challenge
- Chamomile: moody, irritable; unable to release emotional tension.
- Chrysanthemum: deep anguish about one's life and death; difficulty accepting death and dying as part of the life process.
- Elm: despair about fulfilling responsibilities and expectations.
- Gorse: hopeless, expecting suffering.
- Indian Paintbrush: assists in bringing creative ideas into fruition; when struggling with exhaustion from the intensity of creative work.

- Iris: stimulates and opens the soul to receive creative inspiration
- Manzanita: for making peace with being in a physical body and dealing with the challenges of the physical world.
- Milkweed: deeply depressed, unable to cope with the activities of daily living, wants to obliterate consciousness with food, drugs and/or alcohol.
- Mustard: wide mood swings; feels overwhelmed by a "black cloud" for no known reason.
- Olive: depression that accompanies physical exhaustion.
- Pine: despair about one's own faults and mistakes.
- Sweet Chestnut: "dark night of the soul," extreme despair.
- Wild Oat: dissatisfied with work; unable to find one's life work or direction.
- Wild Rose: apathy when faced with illness or other major life challenges.
- Yarrow: vulnerable to the environment and others; helps to create a healthy emotional "membrane" to filter outer influences.
- Yerba Santa: sadness, especially internalized in the chest area; emotional pain.
- Rescue Remedy™, for physical and/or emotional shock. This remedy combines five flower essences:

    - Clematis: Dreamy, drowsy, not fully awake, no great interest in life. When ill, makes little or no effort to get well. May look forward to death. Acute – typical of shock. Deeper presentation – depressed, even suicidal.
    - Rock Rose: emergency, for cases that appear to be hopeless. Accidents, sudden illness, trauma, violence when the person is frightened or terrified. If unconscious, moisten the lips with the remedy. Can be helpful in the dying process, when someone is afraid, viewing death as total annihilation. Name derives from Greek *helios*, the sun. Restores sun-like forces of courage to the human soul to meet tremendous challenges.
    - Impatiens. Quick in thought and action; wants to complete everything *now*. Difficult to be patient with people who are slow. Prefers to work alone. For acute: anxious to recover quickly.
    - Star of Bethlehem. Shock remedy. Shock of any kind tends to drive us out of our bodies. "I jumped out of my skin;" "I was beside myself." Shocking news, the loss of a beloved, fright follow-

ing an accident. Star of Bethlehem unifies body and soul again so that the natural healing processes can take place.

- Cherry Plum. Fear of going crazy, of doing feared and dreaded things they know are wrong, yet they have the thought and impulse to do them. The soul tries to protect against this fear of losing control by tightening its grip, which only leads to more pressure and stress. Cherry Plum is indicated in these extreme times. Gives mental strength and confidence.

CHAPTER FOUR

General Conditions

The Chinese define health as an ever-moving, ever-changing balance. Rather than a frozen statue, this dynamic equilibrium is like an ice-skater in motion or a bicyclist careening down a hill. Often I think of my own life balance as a roller-skating waitress carrying six spinning plates on her arms. Each "plate" represents a different aspect of my life. The challenge is to keep all the plates spinning while the whole of my life skates (mostly gracefully) forward.

The suggestions in this chapter are meant to support you in achieving healthful balance in your life. As you develop the skill of deep listening (see Chapter 2), you will become more and more adept at choosing the treatments that will best serve you. Each body responds to different medicines. You will discover a range of therapies for each condition, with the understanding that your body likely will require different support than your son or your neighbor.

Even for the same type of illness, your body may require different therapies at different times. The cold you had in July might respond to a completely different combination of therapies than the cold you have in the middle of winter. Continue to listen to your body as the guiding source of wisdom for the therapies you choose.

You will have the greatest success in resolving illness and addressing First Aid situations if you *individualize* the treatment. Please incorporate the suggestions in concert with your own intuition and, when necessary, with the guidance of a physician.

ACNE

Skin eruptions can be painful, irritating and embarrassing. Recalling Chapter Two and "Laws of Cure," skin irritations and eruptions are less serious than internal organ diseases because they are closer to the surface of the body. (Try telling that to a teenager getting ready for the prom!) Treating acne requires persistence and a willingness to make lifestyle changes.

Nutritional therapy

- Reduce damp-forming foods. From a Chinese perspective, an accumulation of dampness and heat causes acne. Foods that increase dampness in the body include cold foods (ice cream and iced drinks), raw foods, fatty foods (nuts, corn chips, fatty meats, cheese) and sweets. Foods that cause heat accumulation include meat (chicken is the most warming), seafood and spicy foods.
- Include more whole grains, fruits and vegetables in the diet. These foods are high in fiber and help stimulate elimination of toxins from the body. When the digestive system is overburdened and cannot discharge waste, the body pushes out waste products through the skin.
- Eat foods that support the liver. Skin health is intimately linked with the liver, which is responsible for removal of many toxins from the body. Liver-supporting foods include beets (root and greens), olive oil, garlic and lemon juice.
- Drink plenty of filtered water, at least two to three quarts per day. Water flushes toxins from the body and moisturizes the skin.

Nutritional supplements

- Vitamin A reduces sebum secretion from the oil glands and encourages tissue healing. This vitamin must be taken at high doses for at least three months to produce an effect. Unfortunately, high doses of vitamin A have potentially toxic side effects. Signs of toxicity include headache, fatigue, constipation, dry or scaly skin, mouth fissures, brittle nails, hair loss, nausea and vomiting. Vitamin A therapy should be followed by liver-screening tests.

NOTE: Consult a physician before beginning vitamin A therapy.

- Beta carotene is the precursor to vitamin A and can be taken at high doses (up to 150,000 IU) without risk of side effects. Unfortunately, beta carotene does not have the effect of reducing sebum production but will encourage healing of skin tissue.
- Vitamin E also encourages skin healing and acts as an antioxidant, preventing lipid oxidation and cell damage. Take 400 IU per day.
- Zinc stimulates immune function, promotes skin healing and acts as an antioxidant. Take 50 to 60 mg per day.
- Vitamin C has many functions, chief among them being antioxidant activity and connective-tissue healing. Only four mammals—guinea pigs, fruit bats, primates and humans—do not produce their own vitamin C internally and must rely on their food supply to obtain it. Most humans need far more than the 60 mg of vitamin C that is listed as the Recommended Daily Allowance. For acne treatment, take at least one gram of vitamin C three times per day. See the adrenal fatigue section below for more information about vitamin C.

CAUTION: If you have a history of kidney stones, be sure to drink plenty of water with vitamin C therapy, at least two to three quarts of filtered water per day. Whether or not you have kidney stones, *use buffered vitamin C preparations*. Never suddenly discontinue vitamin C supplementation. Instead, gradually reduce your dosage over at least two weeks.

Physical therapies

- Avoid harsh soaps and ointments that contain sulfur. These cause excessive drying and can irritate the skin.
- Wash the face at least twice per day with a washcloth to stimulate the removal of dead skin.
- Alternate hot and cold applications to the face to stimulate circulation and encourage healing (see Chapter 2, "Hydrotherapy" section). Add Calendula succus (fresh plant extract) to the cold-water application.
- Avoid picking at the pimples and blackheads. Squeezing and picking can cause scarring and further tissue irritation.

Botanical medicines

The following herbal tea encourages liver health and skin healing. Drink 3-4 cups of herbal tea per day, or 2 dropperfuls of tincture 4 times per day.

Combine:

- dandelion root (*Taraxacum officinalis*)—2 parts, by weight
- yellow dock (*Rumex crispus*)—1 part
- red clover blossoms (*Trifolium pratens*)—1 part
- Oregon grape root (*Berberis aquafolium*) — 1 part
- nettles (*Urtica urens*)—1 part
- licorice (*Glycerrhiza glabra*)—1/2 part

Homeopathic remedies

Consult with a homeopathic practitioner to determine the best remedy for you. Generally, a constitutional remedy is more helpful than a prescription based on acute acne symptoms.

When to consult a physician

- If acne persists, despite following the preceding therapeutic guidelines for at least three months
- If acne scars the face
- If acne appears after adolescence, or persists after 20 years of age

ADRENAL FATIGUE

The adrenal glands respond to stress, whether the "threat" is real or imagined. The adrenal glands produce epinephrine, norepinephrine ("adrenaline") and a host of other hormones when you are under stress. Whether you are being chased by a bear in the woods or reacting to a blaring horn in traffic or an angry boss, the adrenal glands respond in the same way.

Initially, when the adrenal glands are activated, both cortisol and DHEA levels rise. These hormones increase blood sugar levels and speed the heart rate to give the body the needed energy to respond to an "attack." In addition, blood is shunted from the digestive tract to the muscles, lungs and heart, to prepare us to fight or run away.

Our ancestors used this dump of adrenal hormones when they fought or ran away. Most of us in this day and age, however, do not respond to stress by moving. Instead we sit in the car, marooned in a traffic jam, or obediently sit at our desk.

The body needs movement to "use up" these stress-related hormones. Because we sit still, the hormones continue to surge in the circulatory system until we finally burn them up by exercising.

When adrenal hormones are running high, we may experience increased heart rate, increased breathing rate, nervousness and sugar cravings (from blood sugar levels spiking up and down). In this initial stage of adrenal stress, vigorous exercise is very helpful to "use up" the adrenal hormones and decrease physical symptoms.

If stress continues over a period of time, the adrenal glands tire. Cortisol generally remains elevated, while DHEA levels drop. Blood sugar dysregulation (hypo- and/or hyper-glycemia) becomes more common. In this stage, moderate exercise is helpful. Frequent, vigorous exercise further depletes the adrenal glands.

In the last stages of adrenal fatigue, both cortisol and DHEA levels are low. In this situation, *gentle* exercise is indicated, e.g., yoga, qigong, tai chi, or other restorative forms of physical movement. Slow, rhythmic exercise, e.g., meditative walking, helps to restore the nervous system as well as the adrenal glands. Over-doing, trying to "push through" fatigue, will only further damage the adrenal glands.

NOTE: Conventional medicine does not recognize adrenal fatigue as a valid condition or "disease." Your family doctor likely will test you for Addison's disease, which is complete adrenal failure. If you test negative, your doctor will likely say, "You're fine!"

In truth, adrenal function is a spectrum, with adrenal health at one end and adrenal failure at the other. The gray zone between these two extremes is the territory of "adrenal fatigue." Conventional medicine considers anything along that spectrum, from adrenal health all the way to the point of complete adrenal failure, as "health." In other words, your family physician will likely miss the nuances of adrenal fatigue.

Testing adrenal function

Ideally, you would test cortisol four times over the course of a day. Cortisol has a diurnal pattern, with peak production from 7-to-9 a.m. Cortisol drops throughout the day, until it reaches its lowest ebb around midnight. Having a one-time cortisol test gives very little information about adrenal health.

DHEA is produced at a steady rate in the adrenal glands. This important adrenal hormone can be tested once, since the levels generally do not fluctuate throughout the day.

Saliva versus blood testing

Blood levels of adrenal steroid hormones check the protein-bound, *inactive* levels of the hormones. Steroid hormones are fat-based hormones and must be attached to a protein to dissolve in blood serum. With a protein attached, these hormones are inactive; they are in their "storage form."

In contrast, saliva levels check the unbound, free, *active* levels of the hormones. I am more interested in the active levels of the hormones than what is in storage.

A simple analogy: Think of the blood levels of steroid hormones as stored food in the "pantry," i.e., fuel waiting to be used. Saliva levels test the active levels of the hormones, i.e., what is actually being "eaten" at the table.

For more information about testing adrenal hormones visit *http://drjudithboice.3dcartstores.com/Adrenal-Profile_c_19.html.*

How to support adrenal glands

The following six steps are an additive approach to supporting adrenal function, i.e., the more severe your adrenal fatigue is, the more steps you will need to incorporate to restore adrenal function.

1　Take regular relaxation breaks during the day
2　Exercise regularly.
  a　In early stage adrenal fatigue, vigorous, aerobic exercise is helpful.
  b　In late stage adrenal fatigue, aggressive exercise can worsen symptoms; qigong, yoga and slow walking are more appropriate.
3　Stabilize blood sugar levels
4　Increase vitamin C and B-vitamins
5　Supplement adaptogen herbs
6　Take prescribed adrenal hormones (DHEA, cortisol)

Relaxation

We have three nervous systems that run all the time in the body:

- **Autonomic nervous system** regulates our heart rate, breathing and immune system, functions we usually do not consciously control.
- When the **parasympathetic nervous system** predominates, the eyes dilate, breathing and heart rate slow and blood flows into the digestive tract. The body engages in significant tissue repair only when the parasympathetic nervous system is dominant. Trying to regenerate the body while the sympathetic nervous system is dominant is like trying to repair an engine while it is running.
- **Sympathetic nervous system** dominates when we are under stress, preparing either to fight or run away (the "fight or flight" response). The

body does not differentiate whether the "stressor" is a bear chasing us in the woods or an angry boss; it responds the same way. When the sympathetic nervous system is dominant, the body shunts blood away from the digestive tract and toward the muscles, heart and lungs, preparing to fight or run away. The adrenal glands make several stress-related hormones that mediate these sympathetic nervous system responses.

Relaxation is your best medicine

All the fancy pills in the world cannot take the place of relaxation in restoring adrenal function. Relaxation truly is your greatest ally in rebuilding the adrenal glands.

Although both the sympathetic and parasympathetic nervous systems are always running, one or the other dominates. I think of them as a teeter-totter, with one side in the "up" position.

The more often you tip the "teeter-totter" in favor of the parasympathetic nervous system, the less you will stress the adrenal glands. When you relax, the parasympathetic nervous system predominates, encouraging

- tissue repair throughout the body
- lower blood pressure
- slower breathing rate
- reduced anxiety
- improved digestion

Many people assume they are simply born with (or without) the ability to relax. In truth, though, relaxation is a skill that can be cultivated, just like swimming, golfing or tennis. Yes, some are born with more talent than others, but all of us can learn.

The simplest, quickest method for shifting from sympathetic to parasympathetic dominance is *deep breathing*. Think of deep breathing as a medicine, something that you "take" periodically throughout the day. Place your hands on your lower belly and feel your hands lift and expand as you fill the lower abdomen with breath. Allow that breath to fill the ribs and upper abdomen and finally the chest. Exhale in the same order: Feel the lower abdomen empty, then the upper abdomen and finally the chest.

Another extremely simple and also deeply effective method for supporting relaxation is to count your breaths. When you are in a quiet, uninterrupted space, count "one" with the first inhalation, "two" with the second inhalation, up to the number 10, or whatever number you choose; then, start over again. This deceptively simple exercise deeply calms our mind and body.

You can also find a simple, very effective guided relaxation on my Web site at *www.drjudithboice.com/relaxation*. Although you can use this guided relaxation at any time, this recording is especially wonderful to listen to at bedtime to relax completely as you fall asleep. Many of us are tense even while sleeping. Relaxing before falling asleep helps you have a more restful, restorative night's sleep. You can also use the guided relaxation if you frequently wake in the night to help you return to sleep.

Steady your blood sugar levels

When blood sugar runs high, the pancreas releases insulin into the bloodstream. Often the pancreas over-reacts, producing too much insulin and blood sugar levels plummet. When blood sugar is low, the *adrenal glands* go into action, producing a range of what are called "glucocorticoids," hormones that increase and stabilize blood sugar. The more your blood sugar fluctuates, the more both the pancreas and the adrenal glands have to work. The following suggestions can help you get off the blood sugar roller coaster:

- Eliminate sugar and simple carbohydrates that spike the blood sugar.
- Eliminate caffeine, which causes the same spike and drop in blood sugar
- Eat protein every two-to-three hours. You don't need to eat a chicken breast or a 12-ounce steak every three hours. Instead, eat a small bowl of bean soup, six almonds and an apple, or half a sandwich.
- Eat foods low on the glycemic index (GI). The glycemic index measures how quickly the carbohydrate in a food enters the bloodstream as blood sugar. The higher the rating, the quicker that food races into the bloodstream as blood sugar, thus spiking overall blood sugar. Low glycemic index carbohydrates that *stabilize* blood sugar include beans, cherries, apples and nuts. High glycemic index foods that *spike* blood sugar include carrots, instant mashed potatoes, honey and parsnips. You can moderate these foods' tendency to spike blood sugar by combining them with low-glycemic index foods. Carrots, for example, could be eaten with lentil soup or fish.

Appropriate exercise supports adrenal health

In early stages of adrenal fatigue, aggressive exercise can be very helpful. *The only way we metabolize these stress-related hormones is to MOVE.* Adrenalin will continue to circulate in the bloodstream until we finally "use up" the hormones by vigorously exercising.

In later-stage adrenal fatigue, the body needs *gentle* movement. Aggressive exercise will strain the adrenals even more, further increasing adrenal fatigue. More appropriate forms of rejuvenating movement include qigong, tai chi and yoga.

For those with moderate adrenal fatigue, water exercise, e.g., water walking or water aerobics, offers more challenging exercise that minimizes stress on joints.

Increase B-vitamins and vitamin C

The adrenal glands utilize large quantities of B-vitamins and vitamin C. The B-vitamins are important co-factors for the production of many adrenal hormones. Vitamin C is so important to adrenal function that the adrenal glands are the *only* place in the body that stores vitamin C.

We are one of only five animals that do not produce our own vitamin C: fruit bats, guinea pigs, parakeets, monkeys and humans. The more stress an animal is under, the more vitamin C it produces. A medium-sized dog under stress, for example, produces *over 15,000 mg of vitamin C per day!*

To maximize the effectiveness of vitamin C:

- Use buffered vitamin C. If you take more than 1,000 mg of un-buffered vitamin C per day, you can acidify the body too much.
- Increase your daily intake of vitamin C to a minimum of 4,000-to-5,000 mg per day. *Please note: People who suffer with asthma should NEVER exceed 1,000 mg of vitamin C per day.* For asthma sufferers, mega-doses of vitamin C increase the activity of certain *inflammatory* pathways.
- Take a maximum of 500 mg of buffered C at one time. Vitamin C is a *water-soluble* nutrient, which means that the body utilizes what it needs within 30-to-45 minutes; *then, it dumps the rest.* If you take large quantities of vitamin C at one time, you will end up with expensive urine.
- Add buffered powdered vitamin C to your water bottle and sip throughout the day.
- *Use a straw*, or rinse your mouth with plain water afterward. Exposing your teeth to citric or ascorbic acid (vitamin C) for extended periods of time will eat away the enamel on the teeth.

Supplement Adaptogen Herbs

Adaptogens are a special class of herbs that help the body better adapt to stress levels. These herbs help support adrenal function as well as the entire hormonal system. The adaptogen herbs also help boost immune function and improve tolerance of extreme weather conditions, e.g., polar cold and/or tropical heat. Examples of adaptogen herbs include Siberian ginseng, licorice, Chinese ginseng and Rhodiola. Consult a qualified herbal practitioner (e.g., a naturopathic physician) to create an individualized formula for your particular needs.

Take prescribed adrenal hormones (DHEA, cortisol)

In mid- to late-stage adrenal fatigue, we may need to take small amounts of DHEA (dehydroepiandrostenadione) and/or cortisol. In almost 20 years of practice, I have only prescribed cortisol once, for someone with extreme adrenal fatigue. More commonly I recommend DHEA, although usually at much *lower* doses than are available in health food stores. Low levels of DHEA can contribute to muscle loss, joint pain, fatigue, sleep problems, bone loss and erectile dysfunction.

CAUTION: If you take too much DHEA, the body converts the excess into estrogen and testosterone. I rarely prescribe more than 5-to-10 mg of DHEA for women or 10-to-15 mg for men.

Work with your health-care provider to discover the optimum dose (if any) of DHEA for your particular situation.

ALLERGIC REACTIONS, HAY FEVER

Hay fever is a relatively mild, although very uncomfortable, form of allergic reaction. Treatment of hay fever should begin at least half a year before the onset of allergy season. Supportive therapies may include dietary changes, nutritional supplements, herbal preparations and stress reduction so that the body's immune system is in optimal condition when hay-fever season arrives.

Mild to moderate allergic reactions may manifest in a variety of ways, from minor headaches or digestive disturbances to itchy, blotchy skin rashes. Severe allergic reactions, called "anaphylactic shock," cause swelling of the airways. Sufferers often gasp and wheeze, trying to get air through the swollen passageways. In very severe cases, the airway can become completely blocked, causing respiratory arrest.

The following suggestions are for hay fever and mild to moderate allergic reactions:

- Nettles, in freeze-dried capsules, two capsules every two hours. In freeze-dried form, nettles have been shown to benefit 50 percent of patients suffering with hay fever symptoms.
- Eliminate food and inhalant sensitivities, if known.
- For hay-fever symptoms, reduce or eliminate foods that encourage mucus formation, e.g., dairy products, sugar and alcohol.

Homeopathic remedies: 30c potency, to be taken every 30-to-60 minutes during an acute attack, or twice per day during an ongoing allergy reaction. Stop the remedy once you notice signs of improvement.

- Apis – edema, swelling and blotching of the skin.
- Carbo veg –"air hunger," wants to be fanned.
- Arsenicum album – allergic reaction to food; vomiting and diarrhea, burning pains, wants small sips of warm water. Anxious.

BOILS

A boil is caused by a staphylococcus infection localized in a hair follicle. The body's immune system attempts to contain the infection by "walling off" the infected area, leading to increased pressure and pain. Often a boil will cause sharp, even excruciating pain before it comes to a head and releases its pus and blood. The suggestions below are intended to abort the boil, if caught in its early stages, or to speed the resolution and healing of a ripening boil.

- The skin is the largest organ of elimination in the body. When other elimination systems (chiefly the liver, colon, bladder and lungs) become overburdened, the body will throw off waste products through the skin. Boils often occur when someone is tired and run down; the immune system is overburdened and the organs of elimination cannot process wastes properly. Encourage elimination by increasing water intake to at least two quarts per day. Eat more whole grains, steamed vegetables and other fiber-rich foods that will encourage elimination through the colon rather than the skin.
- From a Chinese medical perspective, boils are caused by an accumulation of dampness and heat in the body. Boils are more common in hot, damp climates and occur more frequently during hot, humid summers. When boils begin to form, avoid foods and activities that will increase dampness and heat. Dampness-forming foods include sugar, dairy products (especially ice cream) and greasy foods. Heating

foods include alcohol, meat and hot spices. Living in a damp basement or a damp climate can increase dampness in the body. Saunas, sweat lodges and steam baths can increase heat in the body.

Homeopathic remedies 30c potency. Take the remedy 3-to-4 times per day until the pain and swelling resolve (early stages), or until the boil erupts and discharges (later stage).

- Belladonna – early stage, when the area is red, swollen and painful.
- Hepar sulph – for later stage, when the boil begins to develop a pocket of pus. Hepar sulph will cause the boil to discharge or resolve.
- Silica – will encourage the boil to discharge. Silica also can speed the healing of a boil that is slow to resolve after discharge.

Hydrotherapy

You can increase circulation to the affected area, thus encouraging the boil to come to a head, by alternating hot and cold wet towels to the area. Cover the area with a hot wet towel for five minutes, followed by a cold wet towel for one minute. Alternate the towels at least three times. Always end with a cold application. Repeat the treatment in the morning and evening. The hot towels will increase circulation and soften the skin to encourage discharge from the boil. To avoid spreading the infection, be sure to wash the towels after each treatment. Do not share towels with any household members during the time you are treating the boil.

When to consult a physician

- If a boil develops near the eyes or nose, the infection can spread to the brain via the facial artery
- If the boil does not resolve within four-to-five days
- If the boil erupts but does not heal

BROKEN BONES

Broken bones are serious injuries that require medical attention. Get to your primary-care physician or to a hospital as soon as possible. The following suggestions are meant for emergency First Aid, to decrease the trauma of a bone break. Also included are home-care suggestions to speed bone healing.

- Protect the area of the bone break. For a compound fracture (where the broken bone has penetrated the skin), cover the area with a clean, soft cloth. Seek appropriate medical attention.
- Immobilize the area. Further movement of a broken bone, especially of a compound fracture, can increase damage to surrounding soft tissue.
- Research in the early 20th century demonstrated that bones heal more quickly if they are bandaged and allowed to move, rather than being immobilized in a cast, because the stress of movement and weight-bearing stimulates healing in the bone. Although you may not be able to convince your physician to eliminate the cast, you can move the limb as much as possible within the constraints of the cast and request a walking cast for a broken fibula or tibia (lower leg).

Homeopathic remedies: 30c potency

- Arnica – for acute pain, swelling, trauma to bone and soft tissues. Take one dose every 15-to-30 minutes as needed for the first three-to-four hours after injury. Continue taking Arnica as needed until the symptoms resolve. Reduce the frequency of dosing as the symptoms improve.
- Eupatorium – specific for bone pain. Begin taking after acute swelling and trauma have passed.
- Symphytum – stimulates bone healing.
- Calcarea phosphorica – helps reduce bone pain. Calc phos is also available as a cell salt, usually in 6x potency.
- Hypericum – for shooting, nerve-like pain
- Ruta – stimulates healing of the periosteum (surface layer of the bone). Ruta will encourage the final stages of healing, e.g., resolve pain that persists after a cast is removed.

Hydrotherapy can increase circulation and encourage healing. Apply alternating hot (five minutes) and cold (one minute) wet towels to the limb opposite the one that is broken. Increasing circulation in one limb reflexively increases circulation in the opposite limb. This method is especially helpful if the limb is bandaged or in a cast. NOTE: Never apply heat or cold to a cast or splint.

BRUISES

Botanicals

- Cayenne liniment: Add 1 tablespoon cayenne pepper to one cup apple-cider vinegar. Allow to sit for a week. Apply the liniment to bruised areas to increase circulation. CAUTION: Apply to unbroken skin only. Avoid contact with the eyes.
- Arnica oil: Apply on *unbroken skin*, several times a day.

Homeopathic remedies: 30c potency

- Arnica – is the principle remedy, especially for injuries to the head. Take every 30-to-60 minutes immediately following injury, then 2-to-3 times per day until you note improvement. Taking Arnica immediately after an injury may stop bruising and swelling completely.
- Hypericum – injuries to highly enervated areas (e.g., eyeball, hands, feet, genitals) or in case of nerve damage or bruising
- Aconite – hot, throbbing, no discoloration; patient is anxious.
- Belladonna – discolored, throbbing, hot

Hydrotherapy

Alternating hot and cold applications to increase blood circulation.

When to consult a physician

- If you see red streaks developing around the bruise (usually moving from the site of injury toward the heart), a sign of possible infection
- If the area continues to swell
- If a bruise persists for more than 7-to-10 days
- If you bruise frequently and easily (a possible sign of bioflavonoid deficiency, clotting disorder, diabetes, or other condition)

BURNS

Minor burns respond well to home treatment. The sooner you treat the burn, the less damage will occur and the quicker the healing will take place.

CAUTION: Do not apply butter or any kind of oil-based cream to the burn. Putting fat or oil on a burn is like throwing fat on a fire—it will intensify the effect of the burn.

Hydrotherapy

Immerse the burned area in cold water as soon as possible.

Homeopathic remedies: 30c potencies.

Repeat one dose (3 pellets) of the remedy every 2-to-3 hours until pain and inflammation diminishes. Continue to reduce the frequency of dosing until the pain and inflammation completely resolve.

First-degree burn (pain, inflammation, redness)

- Cantharis – for burning pain that improves with cold applications. Also for second-degree burn with blister formation
- Hypericum – for extremely tender, painful burns; shooting, nerve-like pain
- Apis – for stinging, itching pain

Second-degree burn (inflammation, redness and blistering of the skin)

- Cantharis – for burning pain that improves with cold applications

Third-degree burn (charring of the skin, tissue damage)

- Cantharis – for burning pain that improves with cold applications; blister formation
- Causticum – for severe burns, including chemical burns

Botanical treatments

- Aloe vera – soothes burns and encourages healing. The best and cheapest source is fresh leaves from the aloe plant. Open the leaves and use the gel-like substance inside. The skin of the aloe leaf is not effective for treating burns. The second best source is bottled aloe vera, available in health food stores. Look for a product without preservatives. Beware of oil-based creams and lotions, which will worsen the effects of the burn.
- Hypericum (St. John's Wort)—encourages healing of burns. Use crushed fresh blossoms in a poultice. You also can apply diluted Hypericum tincture to the burn. (Dilute one part of the tincture in ten parts water.) Hypericum oil may be used to prevent burns if applied hourly to the skin during sun exposure. For sun-sensitive, fair-skinned people, use Hypericum oil as an emergency back-up only. Hypericum

is not as strong as a sunblock but can be helpful if you are stranded somewhere without any other form of protection.

CAUTION: Do not use oil of Hypericum on burns.

When to consult a physician

- If you have a second- or third-degree burn (blistering and/or charring of the skin)
- If the burn becomes infected
- If pain and swelling associated with the burn has not resolved within 4-to-5 days. (The actual burn, especially with blistering, may take longer to heal, but the pain should stop within one-to-two days.)
- If the burn covers more than 10-to-15 percent of the body

COLDS

A cold is a healing reaction, the body attempting to regain balance after having been affected by physical or emotional stresses. Fever and mucus discharges are a way of ridding the body of external pernicious influences (such as wind, cold and heat—see Chapter 2's section on "Chinese Medicine") and built-up waste. Colds do not require treatment; they are the treatment. You can speed up the healing process, however, by encouraging the body to discharge the disturbance and return to optimal health (see Chapter 1, "Paradigm of Health and Disease").

How To Catch a Cold

Wake up at 3:30 a.m. the day before Thanksgiving to dress. Wake your two young children and herd them into the car. Drive to the airport and park. Stand in the chilly pre-dawn drizzle, waiting for the airport shuttle. Once inside, breathe deeply as you stand in line with everyone around you coughing and sneezing.

You finally arrive at your relatives' house eight hours later and join them for dinner. Eat everything in sight, until you are well beyond pleasantly full. Get into an argument with the brother you haven't seen for three years. Relive every childhood pattern you thought you had outgrown. Stand in the doorway, saying goodbye, without buttoning your coat, for at least 20 minutes. Get in the car, drive to another relative's house and watch football on TV. When dinner time arrives, eat more even though you are not hungry. Besides, you deserve something delicious because your team lost again in the Kumquat Bowl.

This "recipe" for catching a cold includes several physical and emotional stressors:

- Lack of sleep (getting up at 3:30 a.m. to catch the plane)
- Viral exposure (all of those coughing, sneezing passengers at the airport and on the plane; every doorknob, counter and surface you touched in a public area).
- Emotional trauma (arguing with family members; frustration about the ball game)
- Over-eating (stresses the digestive tract and increases metabolic wastes)
- Exposure to cold and damp (waiting for the airport shuttle; standing in the doorway in an unbuttoned coat)
- Fatigue (staying up late after a long flight)

General recommendations for a cold

- Rest! Get in bed as soon as possible and continue to rest for at least 24 hours after the symptoms resolve.
- Stop eating for at least one full day and drink plenty of fluids. Digesting food requires energy that the body might better utilize fighting a viral or bacterial overgrowth. Increasing fluids will thin mucus, making it easier to expel. Fluids also will help prevent dehydration if you have a fever.

Hydrotherapy

- Wet-socks treatment (see Chapter 2, "Hydrotherapy" section) before going to sleep. Begin the treatment with the very first symptoms and you may completely abort the cold. Continue the treatment every night until the symptoms resolve.
- The constitutional hydrotherapy treatment (see Chapter 2, "Hydrotherapy" section) boosts immune and digestive function. Choose this treatment, rather than the wet socks treatment, if you have more time.
- Salt-water gargle—excellent for sore throats. Salt water soothes the throat and kills bacteria and viruses. Add 2 teaspoons of sea salt (better than mined table salt) per glass of warm water.
- Encourage sweating to push out what the Chinese call "external pernicious influences" (EPIs), such as an invasion of wind, heat, or cold. Simmer a tablespoon of fresh ginger in 2 cups of water for 10 minutes, or steep a tablespoon of yarrow blossom tea in 2 cups boiling water for 10 minutes. Draw a hot bath. Sip the tea while relaxing in the bath. Once you begin to sweat, get out of the bath, towel dry and get into bed. Wrap up in warm blankets and allow yourself to sweat. Make

sure that you are not exposed to drafts or chills during this treatment. Your pores are open and, therefore, more susceptible to drafts and chills. In the morning, take a shower to rinse off the sweat and excreted toxins.

CAUTION: Sweating therapy can further weaken someone who is debilitated (elderly persons, or those with long- term chronic illnesses). Also, children usually do not need such aggressive therapy.

Botanicals

- Yin qiao san – a Chinese patent medicine for "wind heat invasion." Symptoms include sore throat, feeling more feverish than chilled, slight headache and yellowish mucus discharge. Do not take the remedy if you feel more chills than fever and have no sore throat—the formula is very cooling. Yin qiao san is meant to cause sweating to help push out wind and heat. Make sure to avoid drafts and chills after taking the remedy. Take three tablets four times per day for sore throat. If you have a fever, increase the dosage to three tablets every 2-to-3 hours. This remedy is for the very beginning of a cold, within twenty-four hours (optimally, within 1-to-2 hours) of the onset of symptoms.
- Hold Echinacea and/or Goldenseal tincture (1 dropperful) at the back of the throat as long as possible, then swallow. This is only for the brave! These herbs are strong and have a local antimicrobial effect on the sore throat, as well as working internally on the cold or flu. Repeat every 3-to-4 hours, as needed.
- Take Goldenseal (*Hydrastis canadensis*) and Echinacea tincture or capsules. These herbs will boost the immune system when taken internally. Take two dropperfuls of tincture or two capsules every 2-to-4 hours, depending on the severity of the cold.

  - Age 6: ½ the adult dosage (one dropperful every 2-to-4 hours)
  - Age 3: ¼ the adult dosage
  - Age 1: 1/6 the adult dosage

Hydrastis has a drying effect on the mucous membranes, making it ideal for any kind of upper-respiratory infection (sinus, lung and nasal). Echinacea stimulates white blood cell production and activity.

NOTE: Some people are sensitive to Hydrastis (Goldenseal). If you notice a skin rash or other allergic reaction developing, stop taking Goldenseal.

- Herbal teas also can help speed the resolution of a cold. Combine equal parts:
  - yarrow (*Achillea millefolium*)
  - blue vervain (*Verbena hastata*)
  - mint (*Mentha piperita*)
  - ginger (*Zingiber officinalis*), dried or fresh

This is a warming tea and may cause sweating. Add 1 tablespoon of the above mix to 1 cup boiling water and steep for 10 minutes. Drink one cup 3-to-4 times per day.

Homeopathic remedies: 30c potency.

Take three (3) pellets 4-to-5 times per day until improvement is noted, then reduce the frequency. Continue taking the remedy at longer and longer intervals until the cold is resolved or until the symptom picture changes. Some people progress through 2-to-5 remedies, each addressing a different stage of the cold. A cold may initially respond to Aconite, for example. If the symptoms do not resolve and the cold progresses, you may move on to a different remedy, e.g., Pulsatilla.

If you are attentive and change remedies as the symptoms change, you may actually be in a greater state of health when the cold resolves.

- Oscillococcinum – Use at the very first hint of a cold, right after the first sneeze. The remedy will not be effective after the first 24 hours. Take six (6) of the small pellets every 3-to-4 hours. You do not need to take the entire tube, as the directions on the bottle may suggest— that is a way of selling you more tubes! Remember that homeopathic remedies act according to frequency of dosage, not the amount.
- Aconite – Take after the first sneeze, when feeling anxious or fretful; symptoms may have developed following exposure to a cold, dry wind.
- Allium cepa – lots of mucus drainage, sore upper lip, excoriating discharge from the nose, bland discharge from eyes; feels worse in a warm room, better in fresh air.
- Arsenicum – affected by changes in weather; thin, painful, burning discharges; patient seeks warmth.
- Pulsatilla – thick, bland discharges, often green or yellow. Changing symptoms: pains move around and do not localize. Patient feels better outside, worse in stuffy room. Wants company, wants to be held (children), improves with sympathy. Best for late-stage, "ripe" colds.

- Gelsemium—slow onset, for colds that begin in warm weather or during a mild winter. Patient feels achy, the limbs heavy, as in a Southern swamp in August. No thirst.
- Bryonia – feels worse with motion, better with pressure. Very hot, very dry, aches all over. Great thirst for cold drinks.
- Nux vomica – very chilly, even while bundled up in bed. Worsens with slight uncovering, or the least movement. Feels chilled from drinking. Aching in limbs and back. Nose stuffed at night. May have upset stomach or other digestive symptoms.

When to consult a physician

- If you have followed the above suggestions (especially regarding rest) and still have symptoms after seven days
- If a child has a severe sore throat—especially if she is drooling profusely and cannot swallow
- If a child has cold and fever symptoms accompanied by a stiff neck or arched back
- If sore-throat symptoms persist longer than three days
- If you have a fever above 102°F that does not respond to the suggestions in the "Fever" section of this chapter

CONSTIPATION

A healthy person with a healthy digestive tract will have one to three bowel movements per day. Normal stools are light brown with no mucus or blood, well-formed, soft and easy to pass.

People suffering with constipation may go two or three days without having a bowel movement. Difficulty passing stools does not necessarily mean you are constipated. The following suggestions will also benefit patients who have daily bowel movements that are difficult to pass.

- Stop taking laxatives. If laxatives are used over a long period of time, the bowel loses its ability to stimulate movement (peristalsis) in the colon. Eventually, the body grows resistant to the laxatives and movement in the colon ceases altogether. During the bowel-retraining time, you may use herbal laxatives 2-to-5 times per week, before going to sleep, to replace the action of other laxatives. Decrease the herbs by half a dose per week until you no longer need laxatives to stimulate bowel activity.

- Increase water consumption to at least two quarts per day. Often constipation results from simple lack of fluid in the digestive tract.
- Eliminate coffee, black tea and other stimulants. Coffee has the effect of increasing gut peristalsis (the contraction of smooth muscle in the digestive tract), but also acts as a diuretic, decreasing fluid in the body. (Each cup of coffee results in the loss of two cups of fluid from the body.) Water and herbal teas are better sources of fluid.
- Increase fiber in the diet. Fiber creates bulk in the intestines, which helps stimulate elimination. The simplest way to increase fiber is to eat foods as close as possible to their natural state. Brown rice, for example, contains more fiber than white rice, which contains more fiber than white-rice flour. Apples have more fiber than apple juice. Focus on whole grains, steamed vegetables and fresh fruits in the diet.
- Develop a regular rhythm for elimination. Some people become constipated because they never make time to have a bowel movement. Generally, early morning is the best time to set aside for bowel training. (From Chinese medical perspective, each organ has a time of day when it is most active; large intestine time is 5-to-7 a.m.) Drink a glass of warm water or herb tea when you get out of bed. Fifteen minutes later, sit on the toilet for at least five minutes. Do not strain or try to force a bowel movement. Get up after five minutes and go about your day. Avoid reading or doing any other activity while sitting on the toilet to ensure that the mind and body associate the toilet with elimination only. Over time, the body will get used to the rhythm and respond with regular bowel movements.
- Never repress an urge to defecate.
- Exercise at least 20 minutes per day, three days per week (the minimum amount of exercise to maintain aerobic fitness). Exercise stimulates colon activity.

Homeopathic remedies: 30c potency

- Nux vomica -"ineffectual urging to stool," never feel completely emptied. Overuse of laxatives. Chilly, irritable.
- Sulphur - frequent urge with incomplete evacuation. Hard, dry, black stools expelled with great effort, pain and burning, especially around the anus. Alternating constipation and diarrhea. 5 a.m. diarrhea.
- Bryonia - dry mouth, dry lips, dry tongue. Stools dry and hard, as if burnt. Thirst for large quantities of water.

- Calcarea carbonica – feels better the longer the patient doesn't have a bowel movement.

Botanical remedies:

- Psyllium seeds – One or 2 tablespoons taken with water or diluted fruit juice after each meal increases bulk in the stool. The seeds are also mucilaginous, helping to lubricate the stool. With any bulk stool softener, you must increase water intake; otherwise, the fiber will bind the stool and make the constipation even worse.
- Aloe vera – Aloe vera gel, made from the inner part of the leaves, is a mild laxative that also helps to lubricate stools. Take one tablespoon after each meal. The skin of the aloe vera leaf is a powerful cathartic that should be used only in extreme situations, not on a regular basis.
- Buckthorn (*Cascara sagrada*) – stimulates peristalsis. Some people experience intestinal cramping with cascara. With long-term use, cascara can have the same side effects as chemical laxatives, so short-term usage (1-to-2 months maximum) is best during the bowel retraining program.
- Senna (*Cassia senna*) – similar to cascara in its actions and effects.
- Slippery elm (*Ulmus fulva*) – helps to lubricate the stool and increase bulk.
- Smooth Move (made by Traditional Medicinals) – a good prepared tea that combines several of the above herbs. As noted above, some people experience intestinal cramping after taking cascara.

When to consult a physician

- If more than a week passes without having a bowel movement
- If you follow the above suggestions and still experience constipation, your physician can test for other causes.

COUGHS

Hydrotherapy

Steam inhalation: add three to five drops of peppermint, eucalyptus and/or tea tree essential oil to a pan of boiling water. Drape a towel over your head and inhale the steam for 5-to-10 minutes or until the vapor begins to cool. Peppermint oil has high concentrations of free menthol, soothing irritated mucous-membrane tissues (which constitute the lining of the entire respiratory tract). Menthol also helps to fight viral and bacterial infections. A steam inhalation at the earliest signs of a cold or flu may abort an illness before it starts.

Essential oils (applied to the chest and neck)

- Combine 10 drops each of thyme, rosemary, eucalyptus and camphorated oil. Dilute the 10 drops of essential oils in 1-to-2 teaspoons of pure vegetable oil. Rub 10 drops of this mixture on the chest and neck 3-to-4 times per day. Stop if the skin develops a rash or becomes excessively irritated. Some reddening of the skin is normal, as the oils will draw circulation into the area.
- Olbas oil, a commercial preparation, also can be used following the directions given above.

Homeopathic remedies: 30c potency

- Antimonium tartaricum - coarse rattling in the chest or larynx. Wet-sounding cough but scanty expectoration. Overwhelming sleepiness during cough or bronchitis. Cyanosis (lack of oxygen leads to blue lips, face, fingernail beds, etc.).Weakened state; end-stage disease. Bronchitis in infants and the elderly, especially in winter months.
- Drosera rotundifolia: Violent cough, severe enough to cause a nosebleed. Turns blue because she cannot catch her breath. Cough is worse after midnight. Cough associated with pertussis (whooping cough). Worse lying down, worse warmth of bed.
- Ipecacuanha (Ipecac): Dry, nagging cough. Coughs so long and hard he vomits or has dry heaves. Asthma with a violent cough. Coughs with every breath.
- Phosphorus – Colds quickly go to the lungs. Worse talking—may have painless laryngitis. Cough so painful patient tries to suppress it. Blood-streaked sputum.
- Spongia - dry, hacking cough, like inhaling a dried, ground up sponge. Barking cough, like a seal. This is the classic second-stage remedy for croupy cough.

CUTS

- Apply direct pressure to the wound, pressing the area with a clean cloth, bandana or T-shirt until bleeding stops.
- Wash the wound with water, or soap and water if available. Washing a puncture wound is especially important, as bacteria can move into a deep wound and remain after the area has healed on the skin surface. Even virulent bacterial infections such as tetanus and rabies can be

aborted by carefully washing the wound. Of course, you cannot rely on soap and water alone. I emphasize wound washing because this simple but profoundly effective support is often overlooked.

- Apply Calendula succus (fresh plant extract of calendula). If the succus is too strong, i.e., causes painful stinging (especially with children), dilute 1 part Calendula succus in 10 parts water. The mixture may be stored in a sterilized spray bottle for use as an anti-bacterial spray. If soap and water are unavailable, applying Calendula succus can take the place of washing.

- Yunnan Pai Yao a Chinese herbal formula that was brought to the West from Vietnam, where U.S. soldiers witnessed its seemingly miraculous effects. The powder can be packed into wounds to stop bleeding, or taken internally. Each package comes with one small red pill to be used only for severe hemorrhaging. The orange-powder capsules, however, may be taken internally—one (1) pill 3-to-4 times per day—to halt bleeding. Stop taking the medicine as soon as the bleeding ceases.

Homeopathic remedies: 30c potency.

Take three (3) pellets every 15-to-30 minutes for acute bleeding. Reduce the frequency as bleeding slows. Stop taking the remedy when the bleeding stops.

- Arnica – helps stop bleeding, especially bleeding associated with soft-tissue injury.
- Phosphorous – for arterial bleeding (bright red blood, usually cascading in spurts)
- Belladonna – helps infection, especially staph and strep.
- Mag phos (Magnesium phosphoricum) – releases muscle tension associated with cuts and other physical trauma.
- Ferrum phos (Ferrum phosphoricum) – helps stop bleeding.

When to consult a physician

- If you are bitten by an animal (wild or domesticated)
- If you cannot completely clean a cut or wound. ("Dirty" wounds, especially puncture wounds, may develop tetanus.)
- If you cannot stop the bleeding with direct pressure
- If infection develops during healing

DEPRESSION

Whenever a patient reports feeling depressed, I always ask if the depression is related to a specific incident (the death of family member, loss of a job, or other traumatic event). If not, I ask if they have been suffering with depression throughout their lives. The approach to depression is very different for acute, situational depression than a lifelong tendency for depression.

Acute depression

In Chinese medicine, each organ is associated with certain emotions. In general, the smoother the flow of blood in the body, the easier the expression of all emotions will be. The liver is responsible for smoothly circulating blood throughout the body. When blood flow is "choppy," we are prone to more physical pain. Stagnant blood flow can also contribute to frustration, depression and anger.

From Chinese perspective, depression is like a swamp. The free-flowing river metaphorically has been blocked or slowed to the point of complete stagnation. The Chinese approach to depression is to support the liver to remove stagnation and re-establish a free flow of blood circulation and, therefore, emotions.

I always warn patients that as the swamp begins to trickle into a tiny stream, the first emotion that often emerges is anger. Usually, anger does not last forever; depending on the severity and duration of the depression, the anger might last days or a couple of weeks. When I prescribe herbs that support liver blood circulation, I encourage the patient to warn his family and colleagues that he might be grumpy for the next week or two.

I explain that anger is preferable to depression. In contrast to the complete stagnation of a swamp, anger requires *motion*. Anger generally lasts for a short period. As the "river" of blood begins to flow even more smoothly, the patient moves on to other emotions, including pleasant ones.

Treatment for acute depression

- Increase vigorous aerobic exercise. Literally moving the blood can help shift the "swamp," or liver stagnation, associated with depression.
- *Caution:* If you have progressed adrenal fatigue, very vigorous exercise can worsen depression. With severe adrenal fatigue, gentle movement is more appropriate, e.g., yoga, qigong, tai chi and meditative walking. See page 100 for more information about adrenal fatigue.

- Chinese herbs that support liver function can help tremendously with depression. One formula in particular, *Xiao yao san*, has been researched and shown to effectively treat mild and moderate depression.
- Increase bitter foods in the diet. From Western perspective, bitter foods increase liver activity and bile production. Greens, such as kale, collard greens and Swiss chard, are wonderful supports for liver function.
- Emotional Freedom Technique (EFT) can be very helpful in working with emotions, including depression and grief. This simple method opens acupuncture channels to allow free flow of circulation or *qi*. From Chinese perspective, this makes tremendously good sense. Remember that where there is NO free flow, there is pain; where there is pain, there is no free flow. This "free flow" applies to emotional as well as physical conditions. For more information, visit *www.EFTuniverse.com*.
- Working with a skilled counselor can help tremendously in working with depression and/or grief. Often the death of a beloved person in our lives triggers re-evaluation of our own lives, on very deep levels. What do I believe? Has my understanding of spirituality and/or death changed? What is important in my own life, in the wake of the loss of my loved one? Why am I here and not him or her? These and other deep questions are a normal response to loss. Taking the time to answer these questions provides a re-routing opportunity in your own life, possibly leading you to a path much more closely aligned with your deepest values and desires.
- Draw on your own spiritual tradition for ways of working with grief and depression. After my sister's passing, an Athabaskan friend gifted me with an eagle feather. She wrapped the feather in black cloth and instructed me to pray each morning, as the sun rose. I would stand at my back window, watching light bleed into the grey sky, praying for my sister and for her easy journey to whatever was next for her. I prayed for my own loss and for the rest of our immediate family, who struggled deeply with her passing. At times my sister's memory would still "ambush" me—I'd find myself suddenly weeping as I dug in the vegetable garden, or crying as a friend described his own loss. With daily prayer, though, my soul knew I had a regular outlet, a time to soothe and re-bandage my wounded heart, so that I had fewer unexpected "blurts" of emotion during the rest of the day. Explore your own spiritual tradition for healthy ways of moving through grief.

- Flower essences can help tremendously during acute depression, particularly grieving. When my sister died unexpectedly, I gave her husband a bottle of Rescue Remedy™, which helped him tremendously in shouldering the grief immediately after her passing. The flower essences do not take away emotions; they offer more ballast to work with the maelstrom of emotions that accompany grief.
  - Rescue Remedy™, for physical and/or emotional shock. This remedy combines five flower essences:
    - Clematis
    - Rock Rose
    - Impatiens
    - Star of Bethlehem
    - Cherry Plum

Notice that each of the following flower essences approaches depression from a different angle. If you have difficulty discerning which essence or essences would best address your particular situation, seek the help of a trained flower essence practitioner.

- Baby Blue Eyes: no longer trusting the goodness in the world; cynicism
- Borage: discouragement, despair, heavy-heartedness
- California Wild Rose: not accepting difficulty or challenge
- Chrysanthemum: deep anguish about one's life and death; difficulty accepting death and dying as part of the life process
- Elm: despair about fulfilling responsibilities and expectations
- Gorse: hopeless, expecting suffering
- Milkweed: deeply depressed, unable to cope with the activities of daily living, wants to obliterate consciousness
- Mustard: wide mood swings; feels overwhelmed by a "black cloud" for no known reason
- Olive: depression that accompanies physical exhaustion
- Pine: despair about one's own faults and mistakes
- Sweet Chestnut: "dark night of the soul," extreme despair
- Wild Oat: dissatisfied with work; unable to find one's life work or direction
- Wild Rose: apathy when faced with illness or other major life challenges
- Yerba Santa: sadness, especially internalized in the chest area; emotional pain

Homeopathy

Homeopathic remedies are very effective in addressing acute, situational depression. Homeopathic medicines offer physical, mental and emotional support. They catalyze the body to go back to normal function, instead of manipulating specific neurotransmitter pathways. Ideally, you would work with a classical homeopath who can guide you in choosing the appropriate remedy (or remedies, over time) to address depression. Some of the remedies your homeopath may consider:

- Ignatia: grief with hysterical sobbing; frequent sighing. Ailments (e.g., headaches, cessation of menses, tremors) with grief or disappointment in a romantic relationship.
- Natrum muriaticum: deep-seated grief with very little outward expression. S/he is closed, refined, responsible and dignified; keeps the sadness of grief and/or disappointed love inside. May be suicidal. Dislikes consolations; prefers to be alone.
- Aurum: deep grief, possibly suicidal. Thoughts of death bring a sense of relief. Hard-working, responsible. Depression from grief, disappointed love, business failure.
- Natrum sulphuricum: Closed, serious, very responsible. May have a plan for suicide but does not act on it out of a sense of responsibility to family. Depression and headaches that begin after a head injury.
- Phosphoricum acidum: Depressed; almost "dead" inside. Physical illness from grief or disappointed love. Mental weakness, apathy; slow to answer questions.
- Arsenicum album: extremely tense, nervous, anxious. Wants to remain in control at all times; plans carefully. Fastidious. Depressed, possibly suicidal, but fears committing suicide. Fears death. Anxious about personal health, about family members. Compulsive disorders.

Chronic depression

If depression continues for more than three months, you are entering the realm of chronic depression. Grief is an exception; a major grief may require a year or more to resolve. If depression lingers for several months, you will need to dig deeper to discover and treat the roots of your condition.

Treatment for chronic depression

- All of the above therapies can be helpful with acute as well as chronic depression.

- Test adrenal function. Adrenal fatigue can contribute to depression.
- Test thyroid function. Thyroid changes, particularly low thyroid function, can contribute to or aggravate symptoms of depression.
- Test neurotransmitter levels. Gottfried Kellerman, Ph.D., has spent the last 35 years developing urine tests to check the metabolites (breakdown products) of neurotransmitters in the body. Urine levels give an indirect, but very accurate, measure of neurotransmitter levels in the body. Think of neurotransmitters as the "hardware" of emotions. These molecules modulate nervous system responses and, therefore, profoundly affect our moods. The testing also recommends amino acid-based supplements that help correct neurotransmitter levels. Amino acids are the building blocks for neurotransmitters and, therefore, help modulate or down-regulate certain amino acids.

  Many health food stores recommend a certain amino acid for depression and another for anxiety. Two people struggling with depression, though, might have completely different neurotransmitter profiles. Trying to take amino acids in this one-size-fits-all approach often will miss the mark.

  The Neuroscience Test gives more specific direction to amino acid supplementation. In addition, the patient *retests* the neurotransmitter levels eight weeks after beginning the amino acids, to make sure they have achieved optimal neurotransmitter levels. This follow-up test helps to evaluate whether dosage levels need to be higher or lower. Conventional physicians are also using this test to evaluate the effect of pharmaceuticals on neurotransmitter levels. The test also monitors the combination of pharmaceutical and nutritional or botanical supplements. For more information, visit *www.neurorelief.com*.

- Psychotropic drugs are prescribed without *any* pre- or post-testing. The prescriptions are based solely on the patient's subjective reports of the drugs' effects. The Neuroscience Test is a wonderful aid in evaluating the effects of psychotropic drugs. Unfortunately, though, many conventional physicians are unaware of the test, or dismiss the 35 years of laboratory experience that have shaped the testing. For more information, visit www.neurorelief.com.

- Take a high potency multivitamin and mineral supplement. Several nutritional deficiencies can cause OR aggravate the symptoms of depression. The B-vitamins are particularly important to nervous system function and moods. Anemia, or low iron levels, can contribute to fatigue and depression.

- Choose "super foods," nutrient-rich foods that provide the body with optimal nourishment. Many struggling with deep depression eat "comfort" foods or no food at all. Appetite often is diminished. When you do eat, choose naturally brightly pigmented foods (sorry, green Jell-O™ doesn't count!) that are naturally high in vitamins and proanthocyanidins, a class of antioxidants that boost immune function, support blood vessel health and improve cellular function.

- Drink plenty of water. Our brains are 72 percent water. Even slight dehydration can affect brain function, compromising concentration as well as moods.

- Avoid caffeine and other artificial stimulants. Although these substances will boost energy in the short-term, they deplete the body's energy reserves with continued use. Think of each cup of coffee or caffeinated soda as a withdrawal from an energy savings account. The caffeine "gooses" the body to put out more energy than it really has. Over time, the withdrawals deplete the bank account; then, we are operating on "credit," or borrowed energy that we pay for in the long run with deeper and deeper states of fatigue. This profound fatigue often drives a craving for more caffeine and more stimulation, which drives us even further into "debt." Get out of debt by stopping the caffeine, guarana, ephedra (now off the market), concentrated tea (Camellia sinensis) and other artificial "energy boosts." They rob us of true, sustainable energy in the long run.

DIABETES

With diabetes, blood sugar runs high and the pancreas does not have enough energy to produce insulin, which helps pack blood sugar into the cells. Those suffering with diabetes literally are starving in a sea of plenty. Blood sugar is running high in the bloodstream, but the body cannot open the cell doors and store the blood sugar unless insulin is present.

Think of the "I Love Lucy" episode in which Lucy had a job packing candy in a factory. She was able to keep up, as long as the conveyor belt delivered candy at a slow, steady rate. When the conveyor belt moved faster and faster, however, delivering massive quantities of candy, Lucy tried to stuff candy everywhere she could—in her mouth, apron and bra.

Similarly, our body tries to "stuff" the elevated blood sugar in every cell possible, particularly the cells that do not require insulin to "open" the cell door to allow blood sugar to enter: heart, kidney, brain, liver and eye. In addition, the body tries to move glucose out of the bloodstream in areas where the blood cools and slows, specifically in the feet, which is why diabetics have so much difficulty with lower extremity blood circulation and healing of cuts or other injuries.

Some diabetics are "insulin resistant," meaning the insulin is present but the cells resist accepting the insulin "key" to open the cell "door." Obesity is one of the major contributing factors to insulin resistance. Often losing weight will reverse insulin resistance and the body is able to regulate blood sugar once again.

Symptoms of diabetes include fatigue, frequent urination (the body is trying to dump excess blood sugar through the urine), sweet-smelling urine and weight loss, usually without trying.

Testing for diabetes

Discuss diabetes testing with your family physician. The most common tests are a urinalysis (which will catch very late stage diabetes); fasting blood sugar (blood test); and hemoglobin A1C, a blood tests that gives about a three-month read on how high average blood sugar levels have been running.

Treatment suggestions

The dietary recommendations are very similar to those given for hypoglycemia. The difference here is that the consequences of veering from your diet are much more severe with diabetes than with hypoglycemia. If you are an insulin-dependent diabetic, these suggestions can help minimize your need for insulin. The less insulin you have to use, the fewer long-term side effects on bone and eyesight you will have. Regulating blood sugar also helps reduce cholesterol formation and end-organ damage commonly associated with diabetes (heart, kidney, eye and/or liver damage).

- The Hemoglobin A1c test is the best to evaluate how well you are regulating blood sugar levels over time. See the section on Hypoglycemia for a more in-depth description of this test.
- Read the dietary recommendations for hypoglycemia. The same foundation information applies for diabetes (see page 148).
- Eating sugar, honey and/or refined carbohydrates is like playing Russian roulette for diabetics. Many diabetics choose to eat anything they want (and often they crave sugar!) and then use insulin to steady the blood sugar. Although this works in the short-term, the long-term side effects of increased insulin use are hard on the body and push you more quickly in the direction of kidney and/or heart failure.
- Eat foods that are low on the Glycemic Index (GI). This scale measures how quickly the carbohydrate in a food enters the bloodstream as blood sugar. The higher the rating on the scale, the faster the carbohydrate enters the bloodstream and the more it spikes blood sugar. Eating low on the Glycemic Index helps to stabilize blood sugar. Low Glycemic Index foods slowly enter the bloodstream, thereby steadying blood sugar levels. See below for the Glycemic Index.
- Not all carbohydrates are created equal! Most diabetes nutrition counselors instruct patients to count carbohydrates. Not all carbohydrates, how-

ever, affect blood sugar levels the same way. Beans, for example, are usually listed among the restricted carbohydrates. Beans help stabilize blood sugar levels for four-to-six hours. Eating pinto beans, black beans, or lentils for breakfast helps steady blood sugar for several hours. In contrast, carrots spike blood sugar levels. Even though carrots are nutrient-rich, "healthy" vegetables, they dramatically spike blood sugar levels and should only be eaten with protein-rich foods, e.g., beans, fish, or chicken.

Glycemic Index of Selected Foods

100%	80 - 90%	70 - 79%
Glucose	Cornflakes	Bread (whole wheat)
	Carrots	Millet
	Parsnips	Rice (white)
	Potatoes (instant mashed)	Weetabix
	Maltose	Broad beans (fresh)
	Honey	Potato (new)
		Swede

60 - 69%	50 – 59%	40 – 49%
Bread (white)	Buckwheat	Spaghetti (wholemeal)
Rice (brown)	Spaghetti (white)	Porridge oats
Muesli	Sweet corn	Potato (sweet)
Shredded Wheat	All-bran	Beans (canned navy)
Ryvita (rye cracker)	"Rich Tea" biscuits	Peas (dried)
Beetroot	Peas (frozen)	Oranges
Bananas	Yam	Orange juice
Raisins	Sucrose	
Mars bar	Potato chips	

30 – 39 %	20 – 29%	10 – 19%
Butter beans	Kidney beans	Soya beans
Blackeye peas	Lentils	Soya beans (canned)
Chick peas	Fructose	Peanuts
Apples (Golden Delicious)		Fresh cherries
Ice cream		
Milk (skim)		
Milk (whole)		
Yoghurt		
Tomato soup		

From Jenkins, D.J.A. Lente, Carbohydrate: A newer approach to the dietary management of diabetes. Diabetes Care 5:634,1982.

- Eating food intolerances and/or food allergies can spike blood sugar levels. See page 31 for more information about food allergies and intolerances.

- Exercise stabilizes blood sugar for a couple of hours. A short, brisk walk after each meal (5-to-10 minutes) helps tremendously in moderating the blood sugar spike that normally occurs after eating. These short bursts of exercise are ideal for stabilizing blood sugar. For cardiovascular conditioning, the exercise episodes should be longer.

- For diabetics, the best time to exercise is *before* eating a major meal. Eat a small snack (e.g., an apple or a few carrot sticks) to increase blood sugar. Walking or other rhythmic activity is a great form of exercise. To better regulate blood sugar, exercise the same amount and the same intensity with each workout. Over time you will have a clear idea of how much you need to eat and how much short- or long-acting insulin you will need to take after the workout. Generally, blood sugar levels are more stable for two-to-four hours after a 30-to-45 minute workout. Make sure you eat a protein-rich meal after exercising!

- Reduce stress levels. When you are stressed, the adrenal glands make cortisol, which spikes blood sugar levels. The more stress you experience, the more difficulty you will have in regulating blood sugar levels. Deep breathing (see Chapter 2) is one of the best ways to temper the effects of stress. Regular exercise will help "use up" the cortisol dumped during stressful events.

- Certain nutrients and botanicals help stabilize blood sugar:

  - Chromium, 1 mg (1,000 mcg) with each major meal
  - Adaptogen herbs. This class of herbs helps stabilize a range of functions in the body, including blood sugar levels. Examples of adaptogen herbs include Siberian ginseng, licorice, Chinese Ginseng and Rhodiola. Be careful with licorice. For certain people, licorice will spike blood pressure. If you are sensitive to licorice, you may be able to tolerate the deglycerrhinated form. Work in conjunction with a health care provider skilled in the medical effects of herbs.
  - Gymnema sylvestra
  - Momardica charantia, or bitter melon fruit

- Address adrenal and/or thyroid issues. These glands must be functioning well to support normal blood sugar regulation.

DIARRHEA

General recommendations

- Fast or reduce food intake until the diarrhea has passed.
- Increase water intake to avoid dehydration, especially in young children. For adults, drink at least two-to-three liters of fluid (dilute juices—half water, half juice) each day.
- Dissolve 1 tablespoon of bentonite clay in a glass of water and drink the clay solution. The clay will draw irritants and toxins from the intestines.
- Eat burnt toast (one or two slices), or activated charcoal dissolved in water. Dissolve 1 tablespoon of the charcoal in a glass of water and drink. The carbon will absorb toxins and reduce fluid loss. NOTE: Activated charcoal will turn the stool black.
- Slippery-elm-bark gruel is easy to digest and soothes the digestive tract. Combine 1/4 cup powdered slippery elm with 3/4 cup water. Bring to a boil and then simmer for approximately 5 minutes. You also can add one or two tablespoons of slippery elm to oatmeal or other cooked cereal. Eat several tablespoons of the slippery elm gruel every 2-to-3 hours.

Homeopathic remedies: 30c potency

- Arsenicum – for explosive diarrhea with vomiting. Patient is exhausted, restless, anxious; desires hot drinks, in small sips.
- Bryonia – following exposure to cold, dry wind, or after a fright
- Chamomilla – diarrhea with teething (infants); grass-green stools with undigested food. The diarrhea has mucus and blood and smells like rotten eggs.
- Colocynthis – frequent urging, severe colicky pains, relieved by pressure and bending double.
- Gelsemium – Nervous diarrhea ("stagefright").
- Nux vomica – diarrhea caused by "dietary indiscretion" (eating too much or eating heavy, rich foods). Diarrhea alternating with constipation. Frequent urging, often with no passing of stool; irritable; chilly.
- Pulsatilla – diarrhea from rich foods and pastries. Diarrhea at night. Diarrhea from taking cold drinks. Variable – no two stools alike.
- Sulphur – Diarrhea drives patient out of bed at 5 a.m. Stools are painless, variable in consistency and amount. Red anus.

When to consult a physician

- If the diarrhea persists for more than two days
- If a high fever (above 102°F) accompanies the diarrhea
- If you see pus or blood in the diarrhea
- If you have severe, continuous abdominal pain with the diarrhea

EYE INJURIES

The major causes of eye injuries include:

- sunburn
- foreign body
- bruising
- laceration

IMPORTANT: Eye injuries are very serious and require emergency care for all but the simplest of irritations.

Treatment for Sunburned Eyelids

Sunburn often occurs when someone falls asleep while sunbathing. This is one eye injury you may treat at home without concern about consulting a physician unless the burn affects the eyeball.

- Apply aloe vera or sliced cucumber to the eyelids. Be sure to keep aloe vera out of the eye itself.

Homeopathic remedies: 30c potency.

Begin taking three (3) pellets – 3 times per day. Reduce or increase dose as needed.

- Hypericum – for redness with extremely sensitive, burning pain; first-degree burn
- Ruta – for burns to the eyeball. Administer while en route to the hospital.
- Apis – swollen lids. Profuse, hot tears. Photophobia (aversion to bright light), but can't bear covering eyes

When to consult a physician

- When the eyeball is affected
- If the sunburned eyelid is blistered or looks charred

Treatment for Foreign Bodies in the Eyes

These suggestions are for care en route to the hospital.

- Loosely patch both eyes, even if only one side is injured. Tight bandaging may cause the object to move deeper into the eye. Loosely bandaging both eyes reduces movement. (If only one eye is bandaged, both eyes will continue to move in response to what one eye sees.) You can use anything for a bandage, although a dry, sterile bandage is ideal. A clean T-shirt or other soft cloth will work in an emergency situation.
- If something is sticking out of the eye, cut a hole in the bottom of a paper cup and affix the lip of the cup to the facial surface (cheeks, forehead, etc.) surrounding the eye, with the object protruding through the hole in the cup. The cup will keep the object from moving and protect the eye from further damage.
- Never put ointment in the eye.

For sand or grit, you may not need to go to the hospital if you are able to remove it by using one or more of the following suggestions:

1. Blink, up to 100 times. Blinking moves objects to the corners of the eye, where they are easy to remove.
2. Flood the eye with water.
3. Push up the lower lid, pull upper lid out and down (over the lower lid), then roll the eye. This will move the object to the center of the eye.
4. Touch the foreign body with a damp sterile cotton applicator (best), or a clean damp handkerchief or bandana.
5. End with a Calendula wash – 10 drops of Calendula succus in 2 tablespoons of water (best to use sterile water or saline solution).

Homeopathic remedies: 30c potency, three (3) pellets 2-to-3 times per day until symptoms resolve. Decrease or increase dosing as needed.

- Silica – pushes out foreign objects

Botanicals

- Herbs to soothe the eye after removing sand or grit: make a tea of Euphrasia ("eyebright") by placing 1 tablespoon of dried herb (leaf) in a cup of boiling water. Steep for 10 minutes, then strain through cheesecloth or other filtering material. Allow the tea to cool to room temperature and then flush the eye with tea using an eye cup (available at most pharmacies). Make a fresh batch of tea each day.

- You can also create a botanical/saline wash. Buy 8 ounces of sterile saline solution, made specifically for the eyes. To make a 1% solution, add 72 drops of Euphrasia tincture to 8 ounces of sterile saline solution. Shake the bottle. Liberally rinse the eye with this solution. Do NOT touch the tip of the bottle to the eye or you will contaminate the sterile solution.

Treatment for Bruises to the Eye

Administer the following treatments en route to the hospital.

General recommendations:

- Immediately apply washcloths wrung out in cold water, replacing as they are warmed by the eye; or apply tofu that has been in the refrigerator.
- After 24 hours, alternate hot and cold applications, five minutes with a warm washcloth, one minute with a cold washcloth. Repeat the cycle at least three times, always ending with a cold washcloth for one minute.

Homeopathic remedies 30c potency.

Take 1 dose of the remedy 3-to-4 times per day until symptoms improve. Increase or decrease the dose as needed.

- Ruta – is called the "Arnica of eye." For acute trauma or for slow healing of the eyeball. After serious injury, you can take Ruta every 20-to-60 minutes as required.
- Hypericum – for sharp, shooting nerve pain and numbness around eye.
- Ledum – black eye. Feels better with cold applications.
- Aconite – sudden heat. Feels anxious. Use during the first 24 hours after injury.

FASTING AND CLEANSING

Fasting—abstaining from eating, drinking, speaking and/or media exposure—can give the body a much needed opportunity to turn inward for healing. Most injured or sick animals instinctively stop eating, to allow their bodies to focus energy on regeneration, rather than digestion.

Cleansing may or may not involve fasting. Cleanses focus on clearing waste from the body. Many companies now offer "cleanse" programs that are simply supplements added to your usual diet. The supplements usually include several "cathartic" herbs that promote bowel movements by irritating the colon (e.g., senna and cascara sagrada); dietary fiber (e.g., psyllium seed husks or chia seeds); and/or bentonite clay, that removes Candida die-off, parasites and mucous from the intestines.

The cathartic herbs are only meant for short-term use, no longer than a month at a time. Initially the cathartic herbs do increase bowel movements by irritating the intestinal muscles and thereby increasing peristalsis, the wave-like movement of the digestive system muscles that eventually causes a bowel movement. Too much stimulation, however, can cause intestinal cramping. Even worse, after several months of use, the intestinal muscles stop reacting to the irritation and do not move at all! Taking prescription medications for constipation have the same effect (i.e., *no* effect) with long-term use.

Recent studies also demonstrate that using the cathartic herbs for a year or more causes intestinal melanosis, a condition of increased melanin production in the colon. Melanosis *may* be a precursor to colon cancer. The bottom line: Find other ways than the cathartic herbs for keeping your bowel movements regular.

Where does waste come from?

Our bodies are exposed to thousands of chemicals and other toxic products on a daily basis. We can absorb toxins through eating, drinking, breathing and/or touching them. The soft part of the sole of the foot and the palms of the hands are the most absorptive skin surfaces on the body. They are also the most likely skin surfaces for us to handle or contact toxic products.

Some common sources of exposure include:

- Food additives, e.g., colorings, preservatives and stabilizers (eating and drinking)
- Pesticides, insecticides and other chloro- and fluorocarbons (breathing and touching)
- Petrochemical exposures, e.g., spilling gasoline on your hands; washing paintbrushes in kerosene; inhaling automobile and truck emissions in traffic (breathing and touching)
- Dioxin (the strongest chloro-carbon known) in tampons, sanitary napkins, diapers, pull-ups and adult disposable diapers (touching)
- Off-gassing from plastics, drapes and carpets; chlorine, ammonia and other cleaning agents; pesticides, insecticides and other chloro- and fluorocarbons (breathing)

When exposed to chemicals or toxins, the body clears what it can through the liver and kidneys. Whatever the body cannot completely clear is stored in fat and lymphatic tissue.

Each body has a certain threshold of waste material it can tolerate. Imagine a trashcan representing the amount of waste that particular body can hold. Each chemical exposure leaves a bit of residue in the trash can. Occasionally, I work with a patient who has had one massive chemical exposure that immediately fills that "trash can," or tolerable backlog of chemical exposure. For most, though, the trash can fills slowly, gradually, over time. The body is fine . . . still fine . . . filling more . . . and then suddenly *wham*, the trash can is full and over-spilling. One final exposure, perhaps even a small one, is enough to move the body from "fine" to staggering under the load of toxic exposures.

When your body has more waste than it can safely store, you may experience a whole range of symptoms. Many of the chlorocarbons, fluorocarbons and petrochemicals mentioned above particularly effect the hormonal system. Several act as "xeno-estrogens," chemicals that mimic estrogen in the body. The following is only a partial list. At a glance, you can see that excess waste affects every system in the body:

- Headaches
- Diarrhea
- Constipation
- Uterine Fibroids
- Endometriosis
- Premenstrual Syndrome
- Infertility
- Breast cancer
- Uterine cancer
- Prostatitis
- Benign Prostatic Hypertrophy
- Testicular cancer
- Prostate cancer
- Dandruff
- Foggy thinking
- Learning disabilities
- Convulsions
- Neuropathy (numbness, tingling, hot/cold sensations and/or other nerve sensations)
- Muscle aches

- Joint pain
- Asthma
- Reactive Airway Disease
- Fatigue
- Flu-like symptoms
- Sweating
- Skin rashes
- Vaginal itching
- Vaginal discharge
- Bloating
- Flatulence

NOTE: Many other conditions can cause the above symptoms. Work with a health-care provider familiar with "environmental illness" if you suspect you may have had significant chemical exposures.

Pushing the body too hard during a cleanse or fast can also cause one or more of the above symptoms. If you notice symptoms after you begin a fast or cleanse, slow down the pace of the cleanse or fast. These symptoms are alerting you that you are moving beyond the body's "carrying capacity" (see below).

Failing to prepare is preparing to fail

When you are ready to fast or cleanse, remember that you will want to *stay within the body's carrying capacity*. By "carrying capacity," I mean the body's ability to safely move waste out of storage *and* eliminate it from the body.

Imagine trying to remove trash from a completely cluttered house with all of the doors and windows tightly locked. You might carry loads of old books, boxes, papers and worn clothing to an exit. If you are unable to open the door, however, you will eventually end up moving the clutter back into piles, or cramming it into drawers and closets.

The body follows the same pattern. Trying to remove too much waste at one time overwhelms the exit gates; then, the body is forced to reabsorb the waste once again.

As one of my colleagues says, "All of the exits gates need to be open before you start dumping waste." Those "exit gates" to dispose of waste include the colon (bowel movements), bladder (urine), lungs (breath) and skin (sweat and sloughing of skin cells).

To successfully cleanse the body, begin by supporting these exit gates. To improve waste removal through the digestive tract, do the constitutional hydrotherapy treatment on page 55. Skin brushing (see page 63) stimulates the lymphatic system (our "backup" circulatory system) and supports waste discharge through the skin. Drink plenty of pure water to support the kidneys and bladder. Deep breathing (see page 67) and aerobic exercise (away from heavy traffic!) encourages waste removal through the lungs.

How do I know if my body is ready for cleansing or fasting?

Before you begin to cleanse or fast, be sure that your body has the electrolytes needed to remove waste safely from the body. Electrolytes are the free minerals in the body. Think of these minerals as the "hardware" that removes waste. These minerals also determine the body's acid/alkaline balance, or pH. You can follow the guidelines below to ensure you have the correct pH, which is a reflection of your body's mineral/electrolyte levels.

Continue checking your pH levels at least once a week throughout a cleanse or fast. If the pH is out of range, you need to reduce the intensity of your program so that the waste removal system can keep up.

With fasting and cleansing, "No pain, no gain" does NOT apply. Pushing too hard or too fast damages the body. Your aim is to remove waste as quickly as you can, while still maintaining your health.

Caution: Beware of programs that offer one-size-fits-all directives for cleansing and fasting. Most of these programs offer no "safety net"—no way of assessing whether or not your body can handle the recommended pace. Checking pH levels is an important step for staying within the body's "carrying capacity," so that you can safely, effectively remove waste.

Checking pH levels

Before you begin a cleanse, eat only fruits and vegetables for one day. When you wake the next morning, complete these three tests to determine your readiness to begin a cleanse program. Complete the tests before eating or drinking anything.

During a cleanse, Steps 1 and 2 (the saliva tests) are helpful in assessing your electrolyte levels. Avoid eating or drinking for at least two hours before checking your saliva pH.

- Step 1: Saliva test
  - Check your saliva pH with litmus paper. Spit on the litmus paper; don't lick it. Record the date and the pH reading on a piece of paper.
    - 6.0 or below: This low reading indicates you may have serious electrolyte depletion. Cleansing or strenuous exercise may be too much of a strain for the body. Replenish electro-

137

lytes (e.g., by eating lots of fruits and vegetables and possibly taking colloidal minerals) before considering a cleanse program. Continue with Step 2.

- 6.1 – 6.3: You have some electrolyte depletion, but not excessively low. Continue with Step 2.
- 6.4 – 6.8: very good! Continue with Step 2.
- 6.9 or higher: Stress or excitement may have interfered with the reading. Wait an hour and test again. If the test remains high, you likely are under significant psychological stress. Continue with Step 2.

- Step 2: Electrolyte challenge, with lemon juice
  - Squeeze the juice of half of a lemon into half a cup of distilled water. Take all of the juice at once, swish it in your mouth and swallow. Wait for two minutes; then, begin a series of six saliva pH readings. Wait 60 seconds between each reading. Make a record of each number. At least one of the last three readings must be above 8.0 to "pass" this part of the test.

    - 8.0 or higher: You passed! You have adequate alkaline reserves, which is an indication of good health. If you also passed Step 1, you are ready to move forward with a cleanse.
    - 7.5- 8.0: These are adequate but not great levels. Proceed with a cleanse *only if you also supplement colloidal minerals while you are cleansing.* Move on to Step 3.
    - 7.0- 7.4: You have some alkaline mineral reserves but not enough. Supplement minerals to increase that reserve and proceed only with a very mild version of a cleanse program. Continue with Step 3.
    - 6.9 or below: may indicate a very serious condition. Electrolyte levels are very low. Pursue a cleanse program only under the supervision of an expert health practitioner. Proceed to Step 3.

- Step 3: Urine test. This part of the test is valid *only before you begin cleansing.* During a cleanse, you will be dumping stored acids, so the urine pH usually will be very low. The saliva and lemon juice tests (Steps 1 and 2) are more accurate than the urine test to assess electrolyte levels during a cleanse.

  - Wet a strip of litmus paper with mid-stream urine.

- 7.0 or higher: You passed! After a day of eating only alkaline-forming foods (fruits and vegetables), your body is replete with electrolytes and is excreting the excess.
- 6.5 – 6.9: You have some electrolyte depletion but not serious. Replenish electrolytes (e.g., by increasing fruits and vegetables and taking colloidal minerals) before cleansing.
- 5.6 – 6.4: You have more serious electrolyte depletion. Consider only a very mild cleanse, eating at least 2.5 meals a day.
- 5.6 or below: Your electrolytes are seriously depleted. You probably did not "pass" the first and second tests as well. Focus on increasing fruits and vegetables and working with the constitutional hydrotherapy treatment (see page 55) before beginning a cleanse program.

For more information about a very comprehensive cleanse program that incorporates pH testing, visit *www.ariseandshine.com.*

Fasting For Physical Health

I was 17 years old the first time I completed a three-day water fast. I found instructions in a booklet at the health food store. Thankfully, the program was well-designed. I drank lemon water and took alfalfa tablets, which are a good source of minerals and fiber (remember the importance of minerals, electrolytes and pH levels). With my history of childhood illnesses and dozens of rounds of antibiotics, my body was extremely toxic, even at that young age. Although I had eaten well and had been running regularly for four years, I experienced many detoxification symptoms (foggy thinking, fatigue, headaches, joint aches and muscle weakness).

One of the greatest gifts of that particular fast was learning a healthy way of reintroducing food. Correctly introducing food after a fast enhances the effects of the cleanse. Eating the wrong foods, or introducing them in the incorrect order, can undo all of your hard work.

After a fast, introduce food in the following order:

- Day 1, breaking the fast: Drink diluted fruit or vegetable juices (half water, half juice). Sip a couple of tablespoons of juice every 15-to-20 minutes throughout the day.
- Day 2-3, after the fast: Add fresh fruits (or raw vegetables, if you do not eat fruits).

- Day 3-4: Add lightly steamed vegetables
- Day 5-6: Add grains and bread
- Day 7-8: Add dairy products
- Day 9-10: Add meats, fish and beans

Fasting and weight loss

Many people fast for weight loss. In the long run, fasting is a poor method for shedding extra pounds. Yes, you may drop pounds during the actual fast. With a sudden drop in calorie intake, however, the body slows its metabolic rate to a crawl. The body perceives that it is under siege and slows to survive what it recognizes as a period of famine.

When you reintroduce foods, the body quickly replaces any lost weight *plus* a few pounds. The body wants "insurance" weight to make sure that it can survive another period of deprivation in the future.

Another potential danger of fasting for weight loss is the mental attitude some people develop. In an extreme, fasting can lead to anorexia. Food becomes the "enemy," the source of our body image woes. For someone who is out of control, food becomes one of the few things s/he can master. *Over*-control leads to a twisted relationship with food.

We live in a culture of extremes. North America has one of the highest obesity rates in the world. Simultaneously, we have many people, especially women, who suffer from eating disorders. They are, literally, starving themselves in a sea of plenty.

Fasting from speaking

I have also experienced "fasting" in groups during silent meditation retreats. Although the retreats included food and water, abstinence from speaking brought a profound inner clarity. I recognized how much energy I expended in speaking. The longer the period of silence, the more power my words had when I began to speak again.

Weekly fasts

For 10 years I fasted every Sunday. The exact form evolved over the years. Initially, I drank only water and continued my daily routine. As I learned more about liver function and pH levels, I drank whole fruit and vegetable juices during the day. Even later I discovered the importance of adding an enema at the end of the day or the next morning to assist the body in moving drier stools.

You may choose to fast from food, water and/or conversation. Phyllis Rodin, a 96-year-old friend who has devoted her life to peace and human evolution, spends every Friday in silence. These weekly immersions in silence have kept her inner "batteries" recharged for years.

The following are suggestions for developing your own fasting routine.

- Decide what your fast will include: food, water, conversation, media, sex?
- Make space for creativity, e.g., writing, painting, singing and/or dancing. Often you will have much clearer insight during your fasting day.
- Drink plenty of diluted juice and herb teas. You may need to eat steamed vegetables and small amounts of protein.

NOTE: If you are hypoglycemic or have special health needs, consult with a health care provider experienced in fasting to modify your program. You may benefit most from a media/conversation fast rather than from a food fast.

FATIGUE

One of the most common concerns patients report is feeling fatigued. We live in a culture that demands a fast pace and heavy workload just to stay afloat. Many of us take on more activities than we can comfortably complete. Personally, when stopping to assess what I could release, I discover most of my functions are "required" tasks; I don't have a lot of fat to trim in my life.

First, consider some of the physiological and biochemical conditions that can contribute to your fatigue. These "big picture" conditions are ones you will need to explore with a physician. If you are struggling with any of these major diseases, they must be addressed. Keep in mind, too, that many of the suggestions for working with fatigue will be helpful no matter what illnesses you do or don't have.

Hormonal causes
- Hypothyroidism
- Hyperthyroidism/Grave's disease
- Peri-menopause/menopause (changes in thyroid, adrenal and reproductive hormones)
- Pregnancy
- Adrenal fatigue

Nutritional causes

- Malnutrition
- B-vitamins (Krebs cycle)
- Vitamin C (adrenal support)
- Anemia – iron deficiency and B12/folate deficiency
- Obesity

Metabolic causes

- Dysglycemia
- Diabetes
- Hypoglycemia

Mental/emotional

- Anxiety
- Depression
- Stress, life changes (Life Changes Index)
- Sleep deprivation

Other

- Cancer
- Chemical exposures

Hormonal causes

Hypothyroidism

The thyroid is the "metabolic set point" in the body, determining the "speed" that our metabolic engine runs. When thyroid levels drop, the engine slows. The body now converts blood sugar, which once fueled the metabolic "engine," into cholesterol and triglycerides. Weight gain, increased cholesterol levels and high blood sugar often accompany low thyroid function, as well as fatigue and hair loss.

Most conventional physicians check thyroid levels by testing only TSH, or thyroid stimulating hormone, made by the pituitary gland. Ideally you would have T4, the inactive form of thyroid, and T3, the active form of thyroid, tested as well. Discuss having these blood tests done with your family physician.

Note: For women, the most vulnerable times for thyroid changes are during three major life transitions: puberty, pregnancy and peri-menopause/menopause.

During these periods of major reproductive hormonal fluctuation, other glands in the endocrine system are also stressed, particularly the adrenal and thyroid glands.

For men, the most vulnerable times for thyroid changes are during puberty and again at the time of andropause (the male version of menopause).

Hyperthyroidism/Grave's disease

With Grave's disease, the metabolic engine in the body is like a sports car constantly driving 120 mph, even in the school zone. The body never slows down. Initially, individuals with hyperthyroidism might feel quite energized, as if they'd had a dozen cups of coffee. Often they lose weight and may develop a fine hand tremor. When the sports car has been cruising at 120 miles an hour long enough, however, the engine begins to run out of gas. In later-stage Grave's disease, the "over-amped" feeling is melded with deep fatigue.

If you have either hypo- or hyperthyroidism, your physician, ideally, would test for thyroid antiglobulin. Both over and underactive thyroid conditions can be caused by an auto-immune disease called Hashimoto's thyroiditis. Usually, in early stages of auto-immune attack on the thyroid gland, the thyroid is *over-active* (Grave's Disease). As the disease progresses, the thyroid tires and begins to *under-produce* thyroid hormone, leading to low thyroid function.

Many endocrinologists do NOT test for thyroid antiglobulin, because the presence or absence of an auto-immune condition would not radically alter their treatment suggestions. For me, this information is vital. If someone has an auto-immune condition, I would be choosing botanicals and other therapies that would help to address the underlying immune system imbalance.

I also would not prescribe Armour thyroid or other desiccated animal thyroid preparations, as I usually would for patients with normal immune function. When the body is exposed to animal thyroid, the body recognizes the thyroid molecule as well as the "foreign" animal marker, i.e., cow or pig, depending on the source of the thyroid. In patients with normally functioning immune systems, this animal marker does not trigger any kind of reaction.

In patients with Hashimoto's thyroiditis, however, the animal marker can trigger the immune system into over-responding. With any auto-immune condition, the immune system is already hyper-responsive. Introducing a "foreign" animal thyroid in the body of someone with Hashimoto's thyroiditis is like throwing fat on a fire; the animal-based prescription worsens the auto-immune reaction.

Note: The thyroid is particularly susceptible to radiation exposure. Think of the thyroid like an umbrella in the throat that protects the rest of the body from the effects of radiation exposure. Many of us have, unknowingly, been exposed to radiation.

In the early 1990's in Portland, Oregon, for example, local physicians reported an "epidemic" of thyroid cancer. This sudden rise in thyroid cancer was linked with intentional releases of radioactive steam from the Hanford Nuclear Power Plant in the late 1940's. The Department of Energy acknowledged that it had released radiation on particular days to study the effects of nuclear exposure on a civilian population. Depending on the wind pattern that day, the radiation moved with the wind northward to Spokane, Washington, or west to Portland, Oregon. Forty years later, the thyroid cancer rates in those wind corridors were many times above the national average. We will talk more about radiation and chemical exposures below.

For more information on hypo- or hyperthyroidism, see page 166.

Peri-menopause and menopause

Peri-menopause literally means "around the time of menopause." This is a six-month to 10-year period when reproductive hormones are fluctuating. Some women move through this transitional period with very few or no symptoms; others have every condition in the book and then some. Each woman is unique in how she will make this transition.

Most women during peri-menopause are estrogen-dominant, meaning they have more estrogen than progesterone activity. Estrogen's general message for reproductive tissue is "divide, divide, divide and don't bother fully developing." Estrogen also increases blood sugar levels and excites the nervous system. Progesterone has a lot of opposite, balancing messages. Progesterone tells reproductive cells to divide more slowly and to fully mature. Progesterone stabilizes blood sugar levels and calms the nervous system.

If a woman is estrogen-dominant, her body is receiving more of the estrogen "message" (that's what hormones are—messengers in the body that deliver different messages to the cells, thereby influencing cell activity). Blood sugar levels initially spike and then crash. (We'll discuss this blood sugar roller coaster below when we explore dysglycemia.) Energy levels roller coaster along with the blood sugar. In addition, estrogen goes beyond stimulating to *irritating* the nervous system, which can contribute to frustration, irritation, anxiety and even panic attacks.

Pregnancy

During the early stages of pregnancy, progesterone levels skyrocket. *Pro-* means "in support of," and *–gesterone* means "gestation;" therefore, *progesterone* means "in support of gestation." Progesterone is the primary hormone that helps maintain pregnancy, particularly in the early stages.

Remember from the discussion above that progesterone calms the nervous system. In excessive amounts, e.g., during the early stages of pregnancy, progesterone goes beyond calming to *sedating* the nervous system.

"I'm not eating for two," said one patient early in her pregnancy. "I'm sleeping for two!"

More than once I've had women patients who tested positive for pregnancy report sudden, unexplained fatigue.

Adenal fatigue

Adrenal fatigue – See page 100 for information on adrenal fatigue.

Nutritional causes

Malnutrition

Poor diet is one of the most common causes of fatigue. In our culture, we understand the adage "Garbage in, garbage out" for our computers, but we somehow think we are excused from the same information regarding our bodies. The higher quality nutrition we put into our bodies, the better they function. Fresh, organic, high quality food is like putting high-octane gasoline in the engine; we run much better.

Another sad but important contributing factor is the quality even of fresh, "natural" foods. Our soil quality has deteriorated significantly over the last two centuries, since the introduction of European farming techniques in North America. The destruction of the soil increased exponentially with the introduction of massive tractors, chemical pesticides and fertilizers. Adding these three nutrient fertilizers to the soil, when numerous nutrients are needed to support optimal plant growth, is a bit like refining whole wheat flour, removing 22 nutrients in the milling process and then adding back five nutrients and calling it "fortified." Sadly, the white flour is deficient in more than 17 nutrients. Similarly, chemical fertilizers contribute only a fraction of the nutrients necessary for optimal plant growth. As a result, our food quality suffers. The food can only be as vital and nutrient-rich as the soil in which it grows.

To maximize the nutrient value of your food, choose organically grown foods, which, according to studies, are about 70 percent more nutrient-rich than their conventionally grown counterparts. You will be supporting the health of the soil, as well as your own body.

Most people in this culture could also benefit from taking a high-potency multiple vitamin and mineral supplement. I am biased toward taking a high-potency multivitamin as the foundation of a supplement program, because nutrients are intended to work together in the body. Walking in a field, for example, you would never trip over a chunk of calcium. This mineral would be found in relationship with other minerals. Similarly, nutrients co-exist in foods. The body best utilizes nutrients when they are in relationship with one another. Taking a high-potency multivitamin and mineral supplement also minimizes the tendency I've seen with many patients to have a drawer filled with individual nutrient bottles.

Sadly, the supplement industry and many "holistic" practitioners encourage people to buy these individual supplements, primarily through articles that tout the benefits of the individual nutrient. A lay person reads the articles and thinks, "Oh, I have all those symptoms. I'll get a bottle of that!" Then she reads the next article. "Oh, that sounds just like me. I'll get a bottle of that, too."

These articles provide useful information but miss the mark in teaching people how to assess their overall health and the "big picture" lifestyle choices necessary to support health. They perpetuate the same mentality as the pharmaceutical companies: Take this for that. This pill will cure that condition.

Sometimes a particular nutrient deficiency will cause a particular condition in the body; we will discuss some of these conditions below. Rarely, however, is that nutrient missing *in isolation*. Usually, the overall diet needs to be improved, as well as other lifestyle factors, to increase health and vitality.

B-vitamins (Krebs cycle)

B-vitamins are vital for the health of the nervous system and the adrenal glands. In addition, B-vitamins are vital co-factors for Krebs cycle, the primary cycle for energy production at a cellular level in the body. If even one of the B-vitamins is missing, the complex series of reactions in this cellular "engine" cannot continue. This cellular metabolic engine shuts down and our energy levels plummet right along with it.

Vitamin C (adrenal support)

Water-soluble nutrients, including vitamin C, are usually excreted from the body within 45-to-60 minutes of ingestion. In other words, the body utilizes what it can of the water-soluble nutrients within an hour and then dumps the rest in the urine. Although vitamin C is a water-soluble nutrient, it is stored in one place in the body—the adrenal glands. Vitamin C is so vital for adrenal function that the gland stores its own reserve. Vitamin C also catalyzes a whole range of biochemical activities in the body and acts as an important antioxidant.

Humans are one of only five mammals that do not produce their own vitamin C. The more stress an animal is under, the more vitamin C it will produce. A medium-sized dog, for example, will produce up to *15,000 mg of vitamin C per day!* The current Minimum Daily Requirement (MDR) is 60 mg. We discussed MDR levels above; remember, they are not set for optimal health.

To maximize vitamin C absorption, take small, frequent doses of vitamin C—generally, no more than 500 mg per hour for adults.

Anemia – iron deficiency and B12/folate deficiency

We can develop two major types of anemia: iron deficiency and pernicious anemia. Both types of anemia contribute to fatigue.

Some of the most common causes of iron deficiency anemia are heavy menstrual bleeding and slow bleeds in the digestive tract for both men and women. Another cause of anemia is a nutritional deficiency of iron. In addition to taking iron supplements, the underlying cause of the anemia obviously needs to be addressed.

Pernicious anemia is caused by a lack of B12 and/or folic acid in the body. As we age, many people do not secrete enough gastric acid, or hydrochloric acid (HCl), to digest food well. The "chief cells" in the stomach that produce hydrochloric acid also secrete Intrinsic Factor (IF). This important molecule must bind to B12 in the stomach in order for B12 to be absorbed across the small intestine and into the bloodstream.

If the "chief cells" in the stomach are not producing enough HCl and IF, the B12 will not be absorbed into the body, even if someone is eating adequate amounts of B12 in the diet. In addition to elders who do not make enough IF, the other major population at risk is vegans who eat no animal products whatsoever. One of the few vegan foods that contains B12 is tempeh, a fermented soy product.

Obesity

Carrying extra weight is a major strain on the body, contributing to high blood pressure, joint and muscle pain, diabetes and a host of other diseases. Keeping your weight in optimal range can have a profound effect on increasing your energy. Discussing weight loss is a whole seminar in and of itself. Hopefully, you will glean some ideas from the energy-boosting suggestions below. Many of the lifestyle choices you make to increase energy will automatically support weight loss and stabilization.

Food intolerances and allergies

Food can cause a wide variety of reactions in the body. Most people think of allergies causing hives, or an anaphylactic reaction with throat swelling and wheezing. In truth, though, foods can cause many reactions in the body, affecting every system and organ. Each person has a different way a particular food affects her body.

As an example, tomatoes almost automatically cause my stomach to cramp; eating yeast triggers a vaginal yeast infection and lowers my immune system. Often, within three or four days of eating a major food allergen, I come down with a bad cold. For me, the immune system is my vulnerable spot.

For more information about food allergies and intolerances, see Chapter 2, or visit my Web site at http://drjudithboice.com/foodtest.html.

Metabolic causes of fatigue

Hypoglycemia

Hypoglycemia, or "low blood sugar": see page 172 for more information.

Dysglycemia

Dysglycemia is a general term, meaning difficulty regulating blood sugar. Usually, dysglycemia refers to the transitional time between hypoglycemia and diabetes. Sometimes the blood sugar is crashing; other times it is running high. If someone takes aggressive action during this phase, he may be able to avert the progression of hypoglycemia to diabetes.

Diabetes

Diabetes: see page 126 for more information.

Mental/emotional

Anxiety

Several of the conditions discussed in this chapter potentially can contribute to anxiety—hypo- or hyperthyroidism; low blood sugar/hypoglycemia; estrogen dominance; food allergies and/or food intolerances; and adrenal fatigue. Anxiety is characterized by shortness of breath, increased heart rate, shaking and an impending sense of doom.

Another factor we have not discussed is excessive caffeine intake. For some people, any coffee intake is "excessive." I have a patient who weighs about 85 pounds and has been drinking 12 cups of coffee every day for the last 40 years. In the past year, at age 68, she has developed severe anxiety and shortness of breath. In addition to her excessive coffee intake—excessive for anyone, particularly someone as small as she is—she smokes a pack of cigarettes a day, which likely also contributes to the shortness of breath.

When we discussed her coffee intake, she protested that she'd been drinking that much coffee for decades.

"Right," I said. "And now the adrenal glands are exhausted from being over-stimulated all these years. Think about each cup of coffee like a withdrawal from your energy bank account. Eventually, the bank is *empty* and you are exhausted, shaky, fatigued."

Reluctantly, she reduced her coffee intake by one-half. Her chronically overactive bladder returned to normal and she began to sleep again. She had much less shortness of breath and tachycardia, or racing heart symptoms. She was still on high blood pressure and anti-anxiety medications.

"Fantastic work!" I told her. "Let's keep cutting down until you have NO coffee. Maybe you can get off the high blood pressure medication, too." I explained to her how coffee increases heart rate and, therefore, high blood pressure. In addition, coffee acts as a diuretic, making us dump two-to-three cups of fluid for each cup of coffee we drink. Dehydration can also contribute to elevated blood pressure.

Sadly, she was unwilling to reduce the coffee any more. She preferred her habits to her health. Of course, she can choose just how healthy she wants to be. She dislikes the side-effects of the medications, but she also does not want to invest in the lifestyle changes that would allow her to reduce or eliminate the medications.

Depression

I always ask patients if their depression is related to a specific event, or a lifelong tendency. I offer different types of support, depending on the severity and the duration of the depression. Fatigue is a common symptom with depression, sometimes so severe that the patient simply cannot crawl out of bed.

For more information about Depression, please see page 121.

Stress, life changes

Increased stress levels and multiple life changes can contribute to fatigue and frequent illness. When we are stressed, the adrenal glands make more cortisol, epinephrine and norepinephrine. We react the same way whether the "stressor" is a bear chasing us in the woods, a talk with an angry boss, or a car honking at us in traffic; the body prepares to fight or run away. The body shunts blood away from the digestive tract to the muscles, lungs and heart. For anyone under stress, the blood vessels to the digestive tract constrict. If you already have a sensitive or weak digestive tract, stress levels further weaken digestive activity.

The stress-related hormones also cause the heart to beat faster and blood pressure to rise. These are wonderful reactions for fighting or running. Most of us, though, sit at the desk or continue our sedentary activities. These stress-related hormones continue to surge in the body until we finally move, e.g., in some form of exercise.

Life changes also stress the body. Working with the Life Changes Index, a diagnostic scale developed in 1967 by Holmes and Rahe, I was surprised to learn that even positive changes stress the body. "Changes in getting along with the boss," for example, scored the same whether the communication improved or worsened. Each life change rates a different score. Death of a spouse rates the highest, with a score of 100. The higher someone's score, the more likely he or she is to develop some kind of illness in the next three months.

When I offer patients this self-evaluation, I give it with the understanding that I want them to see the "landscape" they are traversing and the magnitude of change they are undergoing. Instead of rolling over and expecting to get sick, I encourage people to view a high score as a reminder that their self-care needs to be exquisite. High-stress times are precisely when we need wonderful self-care and usually when self-care goes out the window.

Adult Life Changes Index Test

Directions

If an event has occurred in the past year, or is expected in the near future, copy the number in the score column. If the event has occurred or is expected to occur more than once, multiply this number by the frequency of the event.

Scoring The Life Change Index

The body is a finely timed instrument that does not like surprises. Any sudden change that affects the body, including changes in routine – for better or for worse - can catapult your physical body into turmoil.

EVENT	IMPACT SCORE
Death of spouse	100
Divorce	73
Marital Separation	65
Jail Term	63
Death of close family member	63
Personal injury or illness	53
Marriage	50
Fired at work	47
Marital reconciliation	45
Retirement	45
Change in health of family member	44
Pregnancy	40
Sex difficulties	39
Gain of a new family member	39
Business readjustment	39
Change in financial state	38
Death of a close friend	37
Change to a different line of work	36
Change in number of arguments with spouse	35
Mortgage over $20,000	31
Foreclosure of mortgage or loan	30
Change in responsibilities at work	29

Son or daughter leaving home	29
Trouble with in-laws	29
Outstanding personal achievement	28
Spouse begins or stops work	26
Begin or end school	26
Change in living conditions	25
Revisions of personal habits	24
Trouble with boss	23
Change in work hours or conditions	20
Change in residence	20
Change in schools	20
Change in recreation	19
Change in church activities	19
Change in social activities	19
Mortgage or loan less than $20,000	17
Change in sleeping habits	16
Change in number of family get-togethers	15
Change in eating habit	15
Vacation	13
Christmas approaching	12
Minor violation of the law	11

This final chart will give you some idea of how to informally score yourself on Social Readjustment Scale. The higher your life change score, the harder you have to work to maintain high level wellness.

LIFE CHANGE UNITS	LIKELIHOOD OF ILLNESS IN NEAR FUTURE
300+	about 80 percent
150 - 299	about 50 percent
less than 150	about 30 percent

T.H.Holmes and T.H. Rahe. "The Social Readjustment Rating Scale," Journal of Psychosomatic Research. 11:213, 1967.

Sleep deprivation

James Maas, Ph.D., author of *Power Sleep* (Reed Business Information, Inc., 1997) reports that most humans need nine-to-10 hours of sleep. A century ago, most people in this culture did sleep nine-to-10 hours per night. Today, if you told someone you regularly slept 10 hours, they'd say, "Are you kidding? You're lazy!"

According to Dr. Maas, Americans are among the most sleep-deprived in the world. Several systems in the body suffer when we lack sleep. The immune and nervous systems are hardest hit.

When we are sleep deprived, natural killer cells, B cells and other immune system markers plummet. We are more prone to succumbing to bacterial and viral infections.

Concentration and memory also flag. During Rapid Eye Movement, or REM sleep, short-term memory moves into long-term memory. In our natural sleep rhythm, the body enters a major REM sleep cycle from 6.5 hours until waking. If we wake before this major REM cycle period, we miss many of the restorative benefits of sleep.

A sleep study at the Henry Ford Sleep Clinic demonstrated that sleeping one extra hour per night improves concentration by 25 percent. That's a great reward for increasing your sleep!

When I was a first year student in the music conservatory, I stayed up late to finish all of my studies. The next night, the homework took even longer, because my concentration was diminished from lack of sleep. The next night, when I was even more fatigued, the homework took longer; I slept less and progressed even more deeply into sleep deprivation. This chicken-or-egg cycle—lack of sleep and poor concentration causing me to take longer to complete my homework and thereby increasing the sleep deprivation—continued for the whole of the first semester, until I was deeply exhausted.

Changing time zones can also fuel sleep deprivation. After medical school, I took a job that required me to travel all over the U.S. teaching and training. I changed time zones frequently, sometimes as often as twice a week. After 18 months of travel, I was driving with a colleague in a major city. Looking out the car window at the snowy streets, I asked Kim, "Where are we?"

"Oh, 127th and Main," she said.

"No, Kim, what city are we in? What state?"

I knew at that point that my mind and body were deeply exhausted. Even though I loved the job, I resigned six months later because of profound exhaustion and sleep deprivation.

Many parents of young children, especially those who do not sleep well, also become sleep-deprived. Sometimes this is an unavoidable life circumstance. With luck, you may have family or friends who are willing to give you "sleep breaks" to refill your sleep deficit.

Other

Cancer

Of course, not everyone with fatigue has cancer. One of the early warning signs of cancer, however, is unexplained fatigue. Night sweats are another indicator. Careful here, because many menopausal women with no cancer have both fatigue and night sweats. Different types of cancer will provide other warning clues as well, such as coughing up bloody sputum with lung cancer, or blood in the stools with colon cancer.

Regular annual check-ups can help rule out major cancers. A clean bill of health for an annual physical, however, does NOT mean you can go to sleep at the wheel for the rest of the year. Call your family physician if you have any new, unexplained symptoms, instead of waiting for your next physical. The earlier you diagnose cancer, or any other major disease, the more likely you are to treat the illness effectively.

Chemical exposures

We live in an increasingly toxic world. In October 2006, *National Geographic* published "The Pollution Within"—David Ewing Duncan's account of his travels around the world, visiting state-of-the-art clinics to be tested for chemical exposures. Never having worked in what most would consider a high-risk job for chemical exposures, he was shocked to learn that his body carried residue of dozens of chemicals. He tested positive for 16 of the 28 chemicals commonly sprayed on Midwestern cornfields. Tests also revealed alarmingly high levels of BDH-47, an extremely toxic flame retardant that is now being phased out.

Many of us have chemical exposures, without realizing when or how much we have been exposed. Spilling gasoline on our hands or washing our hands with turpentine after painting is an example of significant chemical exposure. The palms of the hands and the soles of the feet are two of the most absorptive skin surfaces on the body. Our hands touch all kinds of solvents and chemicals on a daily basis. We can absorb chemicals via three major routes: the skin, through touching or handling chemicals; the lungs, via inhalation; and the digestive tract, through the water and food we ingest.

When the body is exposed to chemicals, the liver breaks down and excretes most of the chemicals. What the liver cannot metabolize is stored in fat and lymphatic tissue. Over time, we accumulate a backlog of these chemical exposures. Rarely, I have a patient who clearly had one massive chemical exposure. One, for example, lived down the street from a paint factory that caught on fire, exposing the entire neighborhood to an extremely toxic combination of incinerated chemicals. More frequently, people have small exposures that accumulate over time.

Each of us has a particular amount of chemical exposure we can tolerate. One analogy is an internal "trash can," representing the amount of chemical backlog we can safely tolerate. Once that trash can is filled, either by repeated small exposures or by one massive exposure, the body becomes symptomatic.

Most of the chemicals we are exposed to on a regular basis are heavy metals, solvents, petrochemicals, chlorocarbons and fluorocarbons. These chemicals mimic estrogen in the body. Biologists call them endocrine modulators, or "gender benders." These chemicals won't change a man into a woman. They will, however, dramatically affect reproductive tissues.

Most of our reproductive tissues, in men and women, are made of fat and lymphatic tissue, e.g., the breasts, prostate gland and ovaries. As mentioned earlier, the body stores chemicals in the fat and lymphatic tissue. Because these chemicals mimic estrogen in the body, their message to these tissues is "divide, divide, divide. Don't bother fully developing, just keep dividing." A cancer cell is an extremely rapidly dividing, extremely poorly developed cell. Exposure to these chemicals increases the rate of cell division, thereby edging us in the direction of breast, prostate and/or ovarian cancer. One major cause of the current epidemic of breast and other reproductive cancers is the increasing rate of chemical exposures we endure.

Instead of focusing on cancer "cures," we could avert thousands, if not millions, of cancer diagnoses by reducing or eliminating chemical exposures. The most carcinogenic substance currently known is dioxin, a chemical used primarily in the paper industry to bleach paper white. One simple but effective thing you can do to reduce your cancer risk is to eliminate bleached white paper products, particularly those that directly contact your body. For women, the most common dioxin exposure is from tampons and other sanitary products that are directly exposed to some of the most sensitive, absorptive tissue in the body.

In addition to altering hormonal function, these solvent and petrochemicals also affect the immune and nervous systems. Other possible symptoms associated with chemical exposures are brain fog, fatigue, frequent colds and other infectious illnesses, tremors, muscles spasms, blood sugar dysregulation and a host of other symptoms.

I mention environmental illness because chemical exposure is often overlooked as a cause of symptoms in conventional medicine. Part of the reason for this oversight is that evidence of chemical exposure can be difficult to obtain. The best diagnostic methods involve fat biopsies or specialized blood tests that look for immune globulins for specific chemicals and/or heavy metals. We also have very little research that "proves" the effects of chemical exposures. This research is thwarted in part by our current testing model—the double-blind, placebo-controlled research method which allows researchers to manipulate only one variable at a time. The issue with chemical exposures is that we rarely have just one; they usually come in groups. We have no testing method that can accurately explore the synergistic effects of multiple chemical exposures.

Treatment Suggestions

- If you are in peri-menopause, menopause or andropause and believe hormonal fluctuations are contributing to fatigue, work with a physician trained in bio-identical hormones. If you don't have a local physician skilled in these areas, please visit *www.drjudithboice.com* or read *Menopause with Science and Soul* (Celestial Arts, 2007), which explores the hormonal, biochemical and physiological, as well as inner changes (mental, emotional and spiritual), women undergo during menopause.
- Check adrenal function. As we discussed earlier, if one part of the endocrine system is struggling, other glands may be faltering, too. The Adrenocortex Stress Profile (Genova Diagnostics) uses saliva samples to assess cortisol and DHEA levels. Contact Dr. Boice if you are interested in pursuing adrenal testing: *http://drjudithboice.3dcartstores.com/Adrenal-Profile_c_19.html.*
- Exercise regularly, to support both thyroid and adrenal glands.
- Aerobic exercise improves cardiovascular function and builds endurance. Aerobics also "use up" the stress-related adrenal hormones discussed earlier.
- Early stages of adrenal fatigue improve with vigorous exercise. As adrenal fatigue progresses, however, the adrenal glands cannot tolerate vigorous exercise. Gentle, steady, rhythmic exercise, such as walking or cross-country skiing, are preferable to hard, vigorous exercise for progressed adrenal fatigue. *The adrenal test can help you to evaluate how progressed your adrenal fatigue is.*
- Strength-building exercise increases muscle mass, something aerobic exercise alone cannot do. Each year after age 35 or 40, both men and women

lose a pound of muscle and replace that muscle with 1.5 pounds of fat. You can halt and even reverse this muscle loss by engaging in regular strength-building exercise, e.g., three 10-minute sessions per week.

- Avoid radiation exposure. The thyroid selectively absorbs radiation in the body. Ironically, the thyroid is also highly vulnerable to radiation damage.

- Avoid chemical exposures. Many solvents and petrochemicals alter hormone function in the body. Examples of chemical exposure include off-gassing from plastics; spraying vegetable gardens and/or lawns; using bleach in the laundry; living downwind from agricultural spraying; and cleaning with petroleum and bleach-based products. You can also minimize chemical exposure by wearing gloves when you pump gas for the car or fill the lawn mower; mowing the grass with an electric mower (an hour of mowing the lawn exposes you to more petrochemical fumes than rush-hour in Los Angeles); heating foods in glass instead of plastics in the microwave.

- Filter your water. Chlorine and chemicals can alter hormonal activity in the body. Some of these "gender-benders," e.g., dioxin and PCB's, are also potent carcinogens. The other members of the halogen family (fluoride, bromine and chlorine) can interfere with iodine absorption and metabolism in the body.

- Eat a highly nutritious diet, emphasizing organic foods as much as possible. Organic foods eliminate additional chemical exposure. In addition, organic foods contain an average of 70 percent more nutrients in comparison with conventionally grown foods.

- Eat a diet that is appropriate for *your* body. Eliminate food allergens and/or intolerances. For more information, visit *www.drjudithboice.com.*

- Reduce stress! Although the entire hormonal system suffers when we are under stress, the thyroid gland is particularly vulnerable to prolonged stress. Often thyroid problems surface after a period of grief, prolonged care-giving and/or physical injury. Deep breathing and progressive relaxation are two of the fastest, most effective means for reducing stress. For a guided relaxation recording, please visit *www.drjudithboice.com/relaxation*

- Increase sleep until you have steady energy and concentration throughout the day. Dr. James Maas suggests keeping the same waking time, seven days a week. Gradually move back bedtime by 15 minutes each week. If you currently go to bed a midnight and wake at 6 a.m., go to bed at 11:45 p.m. for a week. The next week shift your bedtime 15 minutes earlier, to 11:30 p.m. Continue this gradual progression of moving your bedtime 15 minutes earlier each week until you have steady energy and good concentration through the day

Many people assume they are rested because they naturally wake at a certain time. This is the *body clock* waking us. The body clock is trained over time to wake and sleep at certain hours. The body clock is set by habit, not by need. In other words, if you set the alarm for 5 a.m. every day, eventually the body clock is set to wake at 5 a.m. That does NOT necessarily mean the body is fully rested.

The body clock also influences our bedtime. That is why Maas suggests gradually resetting the clock by moving your bedtime 15 minutes earlier each week. If you suddenly start going to bed an hour earlier, you probably will flop around in bed for 45-to-60 minutes before you fall asleep. Slowly move back the time you go to sleep to allow the body clock to reset, gradually, over time.

FEVER

Fever is a response to

- endogenous pyrogens (fever-causing chemicals produced in the body)
- bacteria
- exercise
- dehydration

The body produces endogenous pyrogens when bacteria or viruses overgrow in the body. These pyrogens signal the body to increase the core temperature. They also are responsible for many of the symptoms associated with a fever—achiness, fatigue, mental dullness. Again, these reactions can be seen as protective. Often the body needs rest more than anything else.

The body knows that bacteria and viruses can survive only in a narrow temperature range. A fever creates an inhospitable environment for the pathogens. The inability to spike a fever in response to an infection is a sign of weakness and debility. Patients with serious diseases, such as AIDS and cancer, often do not have enough strength to generate a fever. In addition, elderly people may have serious infections without any signs of fever—also a sign of weakened vitality. Diagnosing infections in the elderly and in those with serious illnesses can be more difficult precisely because they cannot run a fever.

Elevated temperature in response to exercise is a normal reaction. In fact, this naturally generated "fever therapy" may help reduce infections during the cold and flu season. Fever due to dehydration, on the other hand, is never a healthy response. If you are working hard or exercising heavily outdoors in a hot climate, make sure that you are drinking plenty of fluids (at least two-to-three quarts per day and even more in a high desert climate).

Prolonged fever, especially in children, can produce brain damage. Serious diseases, however, may result from giving aspirin to children with high fevers. For example, Reye's syndrome, characterized by brain dysfunction (acute encephalopathy) and replacement of organs with fatty tissue (fatty degeneration of the viscera), can result from giving aspirin to feverish children suffering from viral infections. Obviously, not every child with a viral infection and fever who is given aspirin will manifest Reye's syndrome, but the risk of such side effects of aspirin is far greater than the risk associated with high fevers.

Parents often fear convulsions that may result from high fevers, but according to pediatrician Alvin N. Eden, M.D., "a child who has a fever during a seizure does not have epilepsy. Furthermore, simple febrile seizures do not lead to mental retardation." In fact, Uwe Stave, M.D., another pediatrician, reports, "Fever attacks can affect children in quite a positive way. Even though physical strength is reduced, the child may disclose a wealth of new interests and skills. He may find new advanced ways to communicate, think and handle situations, or display a refinement of his motor skills. In short, after a fever, the child reveals a spurt of development and maturation." (Both sources quoted in Rahima Baldwin, "Childhood Fevers," *Mothering*, Spring 1989, p. 36.)

Convulsions rarely occur in children when the fever runs at or below 102°F. The best approach is to work with the fever, keeping it in safe range, rather than giving aspirin or Tylenol to reduce it. Often anti-inflammatory drugs merely suppress a fever; afterward, the temperature can rebound even higher, especially with children. Choosing to use hydrotherapy or other therapeutics requires close monitoring of the child's temperature.

General recommendations

- Drink plenty of fluids (two-to-four quarts per day).
- Rest. Stop your activities and go to bed ASAP.
- Stop eating. The proper translation of the old adage is "If you feed a cold, you will have to starve a fever." Digestion slows dramatically when the body spikes a fever. Food tends to ferment and putrefy, so the best treatment is to fast and drink plenty of fluids, allowing the body to use its energy to support the immune system rather than the digestive system.

- Encourage sweating (if your temperature is below 102°F) to break the fever and push out what the Chinese refer to as "external pernicious influences" (EPIs), which may include wind, dampness, heat and/or cold. Simmer a tablespoon of fresh ginger in two cups of water for 10 minutes. Draw a hot bath. Sip the ginger tea while relaxing in the bath. Once you begin to sweat, get out of the bath, towel dry and get into bed. Wrap up in warm blankets and allow yourself to sweat. In the morning, take a shower to rinse off the sweat and excreted toxins.

  CAUTION: 1) Make sure that you are not exposed to drafts or chills during this treatment. Your pores are open and, therefore, more susceptible to drafts and chills. 2) Sweating therapy can further weaken someone who is debilitated, e.g., the elderly or those with long-term chronic illnesses. Also, children usually do not require such aggressive therapy.
- Continue resting for another 24 hours after your temperature returns to normal. The body needs time to recover fully. If people return to their busy schedules too quickly, they are often sick again with another round of cold or flu within six weeks.

Homeopathic remedies: 30c potency.

Take three (3) pellets 2-to-3 times per day until improvement is noted; increase or decrease this dose as needed.

- Aconite – Hot, dry, cranky. Fever often develops after exposure to cold wind. Fearful, anxious.
- Belladonna – glassy-eyed, dilated pupils; hot, red, dry face; sweaty body; possibly delirium. Sudden onset. No thirst. Specific for strep.
- Ferrum phosphoricum – fever without other specific symptoms.

When a fever goes above 102°F:

- Place a cold washcloth on the forehead.
- Use a cold application (e.g., a bath towel wetted with cold tap water) on at least one-quarter of the body surface.
- Take a sponge bath in cool or tepid water, every one-to-two hours if necessary (especially with children).
- Soak the feet in a basin of cool or tepid water.
- Do not reduce a fever too quickly or too far. Remember, the optimal range for a fever is 99-to-102°F
- Drink a glass of fluid (water is best) every hour.

When to consult a physician

- If the fever persists more than three days
- If the fever stays above 102°F, despite using the methods outlined above
- If a child has a stiff neck, or is arching the back
- If patient has other symptoms, such as burning urination, severe low-back pain, persistent sore throat (for longer than three days), or infected skin abrasions

FOOD ALLERGIES AND INTOLERANCES

Your body reacts to foods in many different ways. Imagine blindfolding a group of people and then asking them to describe an elephant. Each person would have a radically different description, depending on what part of the elephant they are describing. Although the description of the tail is radically different from that of the trunk, *both are equally true and valid.*

In this case, the "elephant" is how your body reacts to food. Each food testing method describes a different "view," a different part of the elephant. Some examples of these different types of food testing are allergy testing (IgE and IgG), constitutional food intolerance testing, ALCAT testing and muscle testing.

Food Allergies

Food allergies can be either IgE OR Immune globulin G (IgG) mediated allergic reactions. IgE food allergies cause "anaphylactic" reactions and generally are quite obvious. Someone with a severe IgE reaction to strawberries, for example, would likely have throat swelling, hives and difficulty breathing within seconds of ingesting a strawberry.

IgG food reactions are *delayed onset* allergic reactions. The body responds with less severe symptoms, from *four hours to four days* after the food is ingested. These allergic reactions are much harder to track, as someone may have eaten the offending food a few *days* before a reaction is evident. If I have an IgG (delayed onset) reaction to tomatoes, for example, I might not connect the headache I have on Thursday with the tomato soup I ate on Monday.

Food Intolerances

Food intolerances are other food reactions *not* mediated by the immune system. Certain foods may cause an inflammatory reaction in the body that has nothing to do with IgE or IgG pathways. Some physicians only pay attention to food *allergies* and do not recognize that the body has other ways of reacting to foods.

Specialized laboratory tests have been developed to assess other types of *inflammatory reactions* in the body. I work with two types of food intolerance testing: constitutional food intolerance testing and ALCAT testing.

Constitutional food intolerance testing

This test assesses the *primary* food or food group that causes inflammation in the digestive tract. They are called *constitutional* food intolerances because *they do not change over time*; they are simply part of the foundation of our body from birth.

Over the last century a select group of physicians has been conducting constitutional food intolerance testing. Originally developed by Albert Abrams, M.D., at the turn of the 20th century, a few dozen physicians in the United States continue to offer the testing. If you are interested in ordering constitutional food intolerance testing, please visit *www.drjudithboice.com*.

ALCAT Food Intolerance Testing

Cell Science Systems offers another form of food intolerance testing. ALCAT (Antigen Leukocyte Cellular Antibody Test) uses a whole blood sample. The test examines the *final common inflammatory pathway* in the body. In other words, the test looks for any and all inflammatory reactions to foods. The test results divide foods into severe, moderate, mild and no reaction. If you are interested in ordering this test, visit *www.drjudithboice.com*.

Why is food testing important for my health?

The better your digestive tract functions, the better you are able to absorb nutrients and discard wastes. If your digestive system is *not* working well, even the best food and the fanciest nutritional supplements will provide very little benefit for the body. From both naturopathic and Chinese medical perspective, *the better the digestive tract is functioning, the better ALL of the rest of the body can function.*

Chinese medicine describes our physical functions more poetically than we do in the West. From Chinese medical perspective, body fat is considered "dampness," which actually makes some sense from Western medical perspective, because fat is a water-rich tissue. Other manifestations of "dampness" in the digestive tract include loose stools, gas and bloating. The healthier the digestive tract, the less dampness we accumulate. A Chinese medical practitioner would support a patient's weight loss by needling points that clear dampness, build the digestive organs and calm the mind (to reduce unhealthy food cravings.) He or she would also likely prescribe Chinese herbs that clear dampness and rebuild the digestive system.

From Western medical perspective, if we eat foods that irritate the digestive tract, over time the junctions between the intestinal cells lose their integrity. Instead of having healthy, tight junctions between the cells, the inflamed intestinal cells develop "gaps," leading to what gastroenterologists call "leaky gut syndrome."

Normally food must be digested to a very small size before passing through the intestinal cells. When we develop leaky gut syndrome, however, larger molecules of food, called "macromolecules," cross through the intestines into the bloodstream. These macromolecules are much more likely to cause allergic reactions.

True allergic reactions are called "food allergies." Often, though, someone has been eating other foods, called "food intolerances," that *irritate* the gut, before developing food allergies.

Common reactions to foods intolerances and/or allergies

Food allergies and intolerances can cause any kind of reaction in the body. Some *common* examples of food reactions include (this is a partial, not an exhaustive, list):

Acne	Eczema
Anxiety	Fatigue
Arthritis	Hay fever symptoms (year-round)
Asthma	Headaches (tension type and migraine)
Attention Deficit Disorder (ADD)	Infertility
Attention Deficit Hyperactivity Disorder (ADHD)	Inflammatory Bowel Disease
Autism	Migraine
Bed-wetting	Muscle aches
Chronic diarrhea	Obesity
Chronic Fatigue	Panic attacks
Depression	Stuffy nose
Diabetes	Urticaria (skin itching, hives)
Ear or other frequent infections	Weight gain

Why do we develop sensitivities or allergies?

Many people unknowingly eat foods they react to. Some of these food reactions are simply part of our genetic makeup, which is why the constitutional food intolerance test developed by Abrams is called *constitutional*. These primary food reactions are simply part of our genetic predisposition.

As discussed above, when we eat the foods that cause an inflammatory reaction in the body, the gut becomes irritated leading eventually to "leaky gut syndrome." Larger molecules of food pass through the intestinal wall and into the bloodstream. These large molecules of food, or "macro-molecules," are more likely to attract the attention of the immune system.

The immune system is used to seeing micro-molecules of nutrients, such as amino acids and essential fatty acids. These macro-molecules of food look like foreign invaders, or "antigens." The immune system creates immune globulins to "attack" these foreign invaders, thereby developing a true allergic reaction.

Eating constitutional food intolerances is often the *precursor* to food allergies in the body.

Other factors that can increase gut inflammation and, therefore, leaky gut syndrome include eating food colorings, preservatives, highly refined food, genetically modified organism (GMOs) and hydrogenated oils. All of these altered foods and additives increase inflammation in the gut. Over time, inflammation weakens the junctions between the intestinal cells and leads to leaky gut syndrome.

Simply removing allergens and intolerances may not be enough to cause the digestive tract to rebuild. Most people with a compromised digestive tract also need to rebuild digestive function. The constitutional hydrotherapy treatment (see page 55) is one of the simplest, least expensive and most effective ways of rebuilding the digestive tract. For more suggestions, please refer to the section on "Inflammatory Bowel Disease" in this chapter.

HEADACHE

Headaches may be caused by a variety of conditions. The suggestions below are meant for acute care, not to substitute for a thorough physical history and examination of those suffering with chronic headaches.

General recommendations:

- Progressive relaxation exercises

Many headaches are caused by muscle constriction and tension. Practice the following exercise during an acute headache and as a daily preventive measure:

Body Sweep

Sit or lie down in a comfortable position. Begin at the feet and slowly move through each body part—foot, ankle, calf, knee, thigh, etc.—noticing any areas of tension. When you sense a tight area, imagine the body becoming warm and heavy there. Continue moving toward the head until your entire body is warm and relaxed.

Once you have completed the "body sweep," imagine yourself relaxing in a favorite environment (by the ocean, in a shady forest or by a beautiful lake). Take a mini-vacation for at least five minutes in this favorite spot. When you are ready, return your attention to the room where you are sitting or lying, open your eyes and take three deep breaths.

- Take a hot foot bath, or alternating hot and cold foot bath, to reduce congestion in the head area.
- Place a cold washcloth on the forehead. A cold application reduces congestion in the head. Combining a cold compress to the head with a hot foot bath will increase the effect of the treatment.
- Rub a drop of essential oil of lavender into each temple.
- Drink lots of water, with a minimum of two to three quarts per day. Many headaches are caused by simple dehydration.
- Increase fiber (whole grains, fruits and vegetables) in the diet. Constipation may cause re-absorption of toxins, leading to "sick headaches." Be sure to increase water consumption so that increased fiber does not bind the stools.
- Eliminate coffee, cola and black tea from the diet. These are common contributors to headaches. Migraines are the exception: Caffeine causes blood-vessel constriction, which reduces early migraine symptoms. (Most migraines are caused by excessive dilation of blood vessels; common headaches are caused by blood-vessel constriction.)
- Tobacco causes blood-vessel constriction. Reduce or eliminate cigarette smoking, tobacco chewing, etc.
- Acupressure stimulation of the following points:
  - Large Intestine 4: the web between the thumb and first finger
  - Liver 3: the web between the first and second toe
  - Yin tang: just above the bridge of the nose
  - Tai yang: the temple area on either side of the forehead
  - Stomach 36: just below the knee on the lateral (outer) side, one finger breadth away from the shin bone
- Keep the extremities (arms and legs) warm.

- Take a brisk walk in the fresh air, being sure to keep the extremities warm (mittens, hat, scarf and boots in winter months).
- Drink red clover or catnip tea at the first sign of a headache.

Homeopathic remedies: 30c potency

- Belladonna—intense, throbbing pain. Extreme sensitivity to noise, light, touch, strong smells. Pain comes on suddenly, usually in the frontal area. Pain may extend to the back of the head. Feels worse after jarring. Face may be red and hot, extremities cold. Pupils may be dilated.
- Bryonia—worse with any motion, even slight movement of the head or eyes. Better with firm pressure to the painful area. Steady, aching pain may be concentrated over the left eye or over the forehead area. Irritable, wants to be left alone. Improves with warmth.
- Gelsemium—heavy head, as if full of molasses. Dull headache. Sensation of having a band around the head. Joints are achy, heavy. Wants to be alone.
- Nux vomica—for headaches following excesses in eating or drinking; hangovers. Generally sick feeling, with possible digestive upset. Aversion to light and sound. Avoids company. Irritable.

HYPO- AND HYPERTHYROID

Thyroid hormone regulates the "metabolic engine" in the body, determining how quickly we burn calories. In addition, the thyroid helps to regulate body temperature, hair growth, joint function, water metabolism and a host of other functions in the body.

Either too much or too little thyroid can create symptoms, some of them life-threatening. As with *any* substance in the body, thyroid has an optimal range, which we will discuss in more detail below.

Symptoms of hyper-thyroidism (too much thyroid production):

- Goiter (enlarged thyroid)
- Warm, moist skin
- Lighter menstrual bleeding
- Jittery feeling, as if you have drunk too much coffee
- Insomnia
- Weakness
- Frequent bowel movements, possibly diarrhea
- Weight loss

- Tachycardia (rapid heart rate)
- Fine tremors in the hands
- Bulging eyes (exopthalmus), eye pain and/or eye irritation

Symptoms of hypothyroidism (too little thyroid production):

- Fatigue
- Weight gain
- Feeling chilly
- Low body temperature
- Heavy menstrual periods
- Joint and muscle pain
- Facial puffiness and swelling around the eyes
- Hand and/or ankle swelling
- Hair loss
- Dry skin
- Soft, brittle, or splitting nails
- Constipation
- Numbness and tingling in the hands and feet
- Thinning of the lateral (outer) one-third of the eyebrow

If you suspect that you may have a thyroid problem, *please* consult your primary care physician. Many other diseases can mimic low thyroid function.

Testing

- TSH (Thyroid Stimulating Hormone): made by the pituitary, TSH signals the thyroid gland to produce *more* thyroid. This is an *indirect* measure of how well the thyroid gland is functioning. The higher the TSH level, the more the thyroid gland is struggling. Many conventional physicians only test TSH levels. We will discuss below why TSH alone may not accurately predict what is happening with the thyroid.
- T4: This is the inactive, "storage" form of thyroid. The "4" refers to four iodine atoms in the molecule. An enzyme, 5'-deiodinase, cleaves off one of the iodine atoms and T4 becomes T3.
- T3: This is the free, *active* form of thyroid hormone.
- Thyroid antiglobulin: This molecule, produced by the immune system, attacks our own thyroid. This auto-immune reaction (the immune system mounting an attack on a particular tissue or organ) is called "Hashimoto's thyroiditis." Most conventional physicians do not test for thyroid antiglobulin, because the presence or absence of auto-

immune disease would *not* change their treatment recommendations. From a holistic medical perspective, however, this is very useful information and guides the types of treatment I would recommend or discourage.

NOTE: In early stages of Hashimoto's thyroiditis, the thyroid gland usually *over-produces* thyroid, leading to hyperthyroidism (Grave's Disease). As Hashimoto's progresses, the thyroid gland tires and begins to *under-produce* thyroid (hypothyroidism). Whether you have hyper- or hypothyroidism, you should be checked for thyroid antiglobulin.

Optimal ranges for TSH

As mentioned above, most conventional physicians *only* test TSH levels, assuming that the pituitary gland is functioning optimally and signaling the thyroid appropriately. This may or may not be a correct assumption. The pituitary can struggle (more about this below) and sometimes the thyroid does not respond to the pituitary gland's signals.

Currently, many physicians are debating the exact "optimal" range for TSH. Some labs consider up to 5.5 a "normal" TSH reading. Board-certified endocrinologists are considering making 3.5 the top of the normal range. Function medicine physicians—those aiming for optimal function in the body—consider 2.5 the top of the normal range.

For those supplementing thyroid, I like to see TSH levels below 1.5. Some people do not feel completely well until their TSH levels are much lower than the bottom of the usual "normal" range. I educate patients about signs of too much thyroid activity (see above, symptoms of "hyperthyroidism") so that we can adjust the dose if necessary.

When working with a patient, I look at the current TSH levels and T3 and T4, if they are available. I'm also interested in seeing what TSH levels have been doing over time. Remember that TSH has an inverse relationship with thyroid: The higher the TSH level, the *less* thyroid hormone the body is producing. If TSH levels gradually increase over time, I know that the thyroid gland has been struggling more and more to produce enough thyroid hormone.

The most likely time for a woman's thyroid gland to struggle is during major hormonal transitions: puberty, pregnancy and peri-menopause and menopause. During these major life transitions, *all* of the hormones are fluctuating, which definitely places a greater strain on the thyroid. Of course, the thyroid gland can falter at other times in a woman's life; these are simply the three most likely times.

Pituitary

As mentioned above, most conventional physicians assume that the pituitary is healthy and functioning normally. Called "the master gland," the pituitary is the feedback loop for all of the major glands in the body: the ovaries, testes, adrenals and thyroid gland.

The entire hormonal system in the body is webbed together. If any of the glands are struggling, you will generally find signs of strain in other glands as well. When the ovaries, adrenals and/or thyroid are going through major changes, the pituitary is likely to be strained as well.

We do not have simple, easy laboratory tests to check pituitary function. The only test we have entails injecting someone with hypothalamus hormones (a gland that "directs" the pituitary) and then drawing several blood samples over the next few hours to see if the pituitary gland responds appropriately (increasing or decreasing its hormone output). Any time a test involves reflexive testing (repeated blood draws after a challenge), the test is rarely ordered.

I know from clinical experience that some patients, particularly women, have had pituitary damage. The most common and easily diagnosed "damage" is a pituitary tumor. Women with pituitary tumors usually begin to make breast milk when they are *not* pregnant or nursing a baby.

Less commonly diagnosed are "sub-clinical" forms of damage, things that would not easily show up on test or X-rays. The most common cause of pituitary damage I have seen is radiation exposure(s).

Interestingly, the thyroid also reacts strongly to radiation exposure. The thyroid selectively "takes up" radiation in the body, acting as screen that protects other organs and glands from high radiation exposure.

Thyroid supplementation for hypothyroidism (low thyroid function)

If you have thyroid testing done and discover you have low thyroid levels, carefully consider what type of thyroid medication would best suit your needs.

Most conventional physicians prescribe Synthroid or Levo-thyroxine. Both are forms of T4, the *inactive* form of thyroid hormone. Remember that the body requires enzyme 5'-deiodinase to cleave off one of the iodine atoms to make T3, the active form of thyroid.

Some people do not make enough 5'-deiodinase. These patients are low in T3 and may still suffer from low-thyroid symptoms, even though they are taking a thyroid prescription.

This decreased ability to convert T4 to T3 is called "Wilson's Syndrome," named after E. Denis Wilson, M.D., who first treated and wrote about the condition. Dr. Wilson developed a special protocol using T3, or Cytomel, to correct the 5'-deiodinase enzyme levels in the body.

Side note: The pituitary does *not* differentiate between T3 and T4 when it is monitoring blood levels of thyroid hormone. That explains why patients with Wilson's Syndrome often have normal TSH levels. Only by testing T3 and T4 levels, as well as correlating the testing information with a patient's symptoms, would a physician arrive at a diagnosis of Wilson's Syndrome.

Many patients who do not respond well to Synthroid or Levo-thyroxine fare much better taking Armour Thyroid or Naturethroid. These thyroid prescriptions are made from desiccated (dried) animal thyroid.

Before 1970, physicians could prescribe only Armour Thyroid. Only in 1970 did synthetic forms (Synthroid) of thyroid hormone become available. Based on clinical studies conducted in the 1950's, many physicians suspected that patients were receiving unpredictable ratios of T3 and T4 in the animal form of thyroid. This research was repeated in the 1990's, proving that T3 and T4 levels in desiccated animal thyroid were much more stable than previously thought.

I usually prescribe Armour Thyroid or Naturethroid. The only exception to that rule is patients with Hashimoto's Thyroiditis. For those already suffering with this auto-immune condition, the animal source of thyroid would be perceived as "foreign," and the immune system would begin to attack the "invading" foreigner. With the immune system on red-alert, the body would produce more thyroid anti-globulin and the thyroid gland would be caught in the crossfire. In other words, the animal source of thyroid could worsen (and very rarely *create*) this particular auto-immune reaction.

For those suffering with Hashimoto's, I prescribe a combination of Levo-thyroxine or Synthroid (T4) with Cytomel (T3).

What about taking iodine to support my thyroid?

A century ago, many Midwestern women suffered with low thyroid function because of a deficiency of iodine in their diet. At that time we did not have the shipping abilities we have today and many people in the middle of the continent did not have iodine-rich seafood or sea vegetables (e.g., seaweed) to eat, especially in the winter. The Midwestern diet also relied heavily on brassica (Brassicaceae) or cruciferous (Cruciferae) family foods, e.g., cabbage, broccoli, cauliflower and kale. In large amounts, these vegetables can inhibit thyroid function.

Remember that iodine atoms are a key component of thyroid hormone, which is why iodine levels in the body are so important. To correct this situation, salt companies added iodine to salt. For the most part, this remedied the situation.

Edgar Cayce suggested taking a purified liquid iodine supplement, Atomidine. This particular preparation of iodine can be taken internally or used externally. For those with true iodine deficiencies, these iodine supplements really helped.

CAUTION: Some nutritionists and health food store personnel will recommend iodine for any thyroid problem.

PLEASE NOTE: For those with Grave's Disease (hyperthyroidism, too much thyroid), increasing iodine can cause a "thyroid storm," or "thyrotoxicosis." During a thyroid storm, the body suddenly, dramatically increases thyroid production. This can cause a rapid increase in heart rate, anxiety and potentially heart failure.

For those with Hashimoto's thyroiditis, iodine can also cause a thyroid storm. This is another reason why I want to know if patients have an underlying autoimmune disease that is driving their hypothyroidism (low thyroid function).

PLEASE consult with someone trained in medical nutrition, e.g., a naturopathic physician, before supplementing iodine.

What else can I do to support my thyroid?

- Check adrenal function. As we discussed earlier, if one part of the endocrine system is struggling, other glands may be faltering, too. The Adrenocortex Stress Profile (Genova Diagnostics) uses saliva samples to assess cortisol and DHEA levels. Contact Dr. Boice if you are interested in pursuing adrenal testing.
  http://drjudithboice.3dcartstores.com/Adrenal-Profile_c_19.html
- Exercise regularly, to support both thyroid and adrenal glands.
- Avoid radiation exposure. The thyroid selectively absorbs radiation in the body. Ironically, the thyroid is also highly vulnerable to radiation damage.
- Avoid chemical exposures. Many solvents and petrochemicals alter hormone function in the body. Examples of chemical exposure include off-gassing from plastics; spraying vegetable gardens and/or lawns; using bleach in the laundry; living downwind from agricultural spraying; cleaning with petroleum and bleach-based products.
- Filter your water. Chlorine and chemicals can alter hormonal activity in the body. Some of these "gender-benders," e.g., dioxin and PCB's, are also potent carcinogens. The other members of the halogen family

(fluoride, bromine and chlorine) can interfere with iodine absorption and metabolism in the body.

- Eat a highly nutritious diet, emphasizing organic foods as much as possible. Organic foods eliminate additional chemical exposure. In addition, organic foods contain an average of 70 percent more nutrients in comparison with conventionally grown foods.

- Eat a diet that is appropriate for *your* body. Eliminate food allergens and/or intolerances. For more information, visit *www.drjudithboice.com/foodtest.html.*

- Reduce stress! Although the entire hormonal system suffers when we are under stress, the thyroid gland is particularly vulnerable to prolonged stress. Often thyroid problems surface after a period of grief, prolonged care-giving and/or physical injury. Deep breathing and progressive relaxation are two of the fastest, most effective means for reducing stress. For a guided relaxation recording, visit *www.drjudithboice.com/relaxation.*

HYPOGLYCEMIA AND DYSGLYCEMIA

Hypoglycemia, or "low blood sugar," is usually the first stage of blood sugar regulation problems. When you eat sweets or other foods that cause a blood sugar spike, the pancreas over-responds, makes too much insulin to move blood sugar out of the bloodstream and into the cells, and then blood sugar plummets. In this low blood sugar state, you usually feel weak and jittery. Some people become anxious, nervous or crabby. In severe cases, you may not be able to think at all.

When the blood sugar plummets, the adrenal glands kick in, producing "glucocorticoids"—hormones that elevate blood sugar. The body craves something sweet or a cup of coffee to spike the blood sugar again. You eat the donut, drink the coffee and feel great for about 45 minutes—until the pancreas again produces a huge surge of insulin, which precipitously drops blood sugar. Many people ride this roller coaster all day long, with their moods and energy levels rocketing and dropping right along with the blood sugar.

If this roller coaster ride continues long enough, both the adrenal glands and the pancreas tire. The exhausted pancreas stops producing enough insulin. Blood sugar levels rise and stay high, without insulin to "open" the cell door and pack away blood sugar. Now the body shifts from hypoglycemia to hyperglycemia, or diabetes.

The best approach is to work with blood sugar regulation during this hypo-glycemic phase and not stress the pancreas to the point of developing diabetes. We will discuss steps to take below.

Other hormonal conditions can also contribute to hypoglycemia. Periods of major hormonal fluctuation, e.g., puberty, pregnancy, menopause and andro-pause, can aggravate blood sugar regulation issues. Both the adrenal glands and the thyroid are prone to falter during these periods of hormonal fluctuation. Low adrenal function (not *failure* but, rather, adrenal fatigue) may contribute to blood sugar regulation issues, especially hypoglycemia. See page 100 for more information on adrenal fatigue. Low thyroid function (hypothyroidism) (see page 166) can also contribute to blood sugar regulation issues.

One patient in her mid-sixties had suffered with hypoglycemia for several years, roughly from the time she entered menopause. If she stretched meal times more than three hours apart, her hands began to shake, her mind was foggy, and she felt very weak. If she regularly ate protein, her blood sugar levels stayed stable and she could function well.

Testing for adrenal function revealed she was in late-stage adrenal fatigue. After more than a year of rebuilding and restoring adrenal function, she was able to stretch mealtimes to four or five hours apart without discomfort.

Ideally, blood sugar fluctuates in a mid-range, rather than rocketing up and down. Our body struggles with sudden increases in blood sugar. The body has to find a place to pack away the surge of blood sugar. The pancreas dumps insulin, which allows the body to "stuff" the sugar in every available cell. Small fluctuations in a mid-range are fine; the roller coaster is not.

Dysglycemia

Dysglycemia is a general term, meaning difficulty regulating blood sugar. Usually, dysglycemia refers to the transitional time between hypoglycemia and diabetes. The blood sugar alternates between crashing, when the pancreas is making too much insulin; and running high, when the pancreas is too tired to produce enough insulin.

Blood sugar testing

Fasting blood sugar levels are measured after at least 12 hours with no food. People suffering with hypoglycemia often have low fasting blood sugar levels, below 65 mg/dl. The "gold standard" test for hypoglycemia is the Glucose Tolerance Test (GTT). Patients ingest an incredibly sweet drink and then have blood drawn five times over three hours to assess how quickly the blood sugar level spikes, drops and/or normalizes.

For someone with severe hypoglycemia, this can be a brutal test. Most clinicians recommend a trial hypoglycemic diet (see suggestions below). If their symptoms improve, the clinician assumes the patient has low blood sugar.

During pregnancy, patients usually are told to eat a certain breakfast, with a known sugar content and then blood sugar levels are tested for several hours after eating.

Hemoglobin A1c, or "glycosylated hemoglobin," gives a longer term read on blood sugar levels. When blood sugar levels spike, glucose alters or "glycosylates" the hemoglobin in red blood cells. When viewed under a high-powered field in a microscope, the glycosylated hemoglobin has a characteristic appearance. The number tells how many altered red blood cells are visible in the high-powered microscope field. The higher the number, the higher blood sugar levels have been running over a three-month period. This test gives a three-month view because red blood cells live for approximately three months in the bloodstream.

The "normal" range for Hemoglobin A1c varies from lab to lab. Some labs consider up to 6.0 normal; others consider 5.8 the top of the normal range. I consider 5.7 or higher a problem. The higher the number, the more difficulty the body is having in regulating blood sugar.

Hemoglobin A1C is an earlier warning system for blood sugar levels than fasting blood sugar. By the time fasting blood sugar levels are elevated, the body usually has passed into the realm of diabetes.

For patients struggling with dysglycemia, Hemoglobin A1c levels usually are right on the border of diabetes (5.7- 6.0).Taking aggressive action during this phase can avert the progression of hypoglycemia to diabetes. Diet, exercise and certain supplements are your best allies in steadying blood sugar.

Treatment suggestions

- Eat protein every two-to-three hours. You do not necessarily need to eat a 12-ounce steak every three hours. Beans, nuts and certain whole grains such as quinoa are protein-rich. Cheese is *not* a great protein source. Think of cheese primarily as dairy fat with a bit of protein swirled in.

- Eat breakfast, lunch, dinner and a mid-morning and mid-afternoon snack. Make your main meals a little bit smaller (e.g., perhaps three instead of four ounces of protein at lunch). Snacks might be half of a bean burrito or tuna fish sandwich, a small bowl of bean soup, or an apple with six almonds.

- Avoid simple carbohydrates, e.g., white flour, white rice and sugar. These foods race into the bloodstream and spike blood sugar.

- Avoid even the "healthy" concentrated sweeteners, such as honey and maple syrup. Although these sweeteners have more nutritional value than cane juice sugar, they still will spike blood sugar levels.

- "Evaporated cane juice" is the new euphemism for sugar—doesn't that sound so much healthier? It's still sugar!

- Eat foods that are low on the Glycemic Index (GI). This scale measures how quickly the carbohydrate in a food enters the bloodstream as blood sugar. The higher the rating on the scale, the faster the carbohydrate enters the bloodstream and the more it spikes blood sugar. Eating low on the glycemic index helps to stabilize blood sugar. Low Glycemic Index foods slowly enter the blood stream, thereby steadying blood sugar levels. See page 128 for the Glycemic Index.

- Beans help stabilize blood sugar levels for four-to-six hours. Eating pinto beans, black beans or lentils for breakfast helps steady blood sugar for several hours.

- Eating food intolerances and/or food allergies can spike blood sugar levels. See page 31 for more information about food allergies and intolerances.

- Exercise stabilizes blood sugar for a couple of hours. A short, brisk walk after each meal (five-to-10 minutes) helps tremendously in moderating the blood sugar spike that normally occurs after eating. These short bursts of exercise are ideal for stabilizing blood sugar. For cardiovascular conditioning, the exercise episodes should be longer.

- Many patients complain that they don't have time to exercise, or the weather disrupts their exercise schedule. During the winter, I keep a small pedal machine in the clinic so that I can exercise for a few minutes after eating. These pedal machines are inexpensive (usually $40-$50), compact and easy to use. Simply sit on a chair or sofa, place the machine in front of you and pedal away. You can also place the machine on a table or desk and exercise the arms.

- Reduce stress levels. Remember that the more stress you endure, the more you strain the adrenal glands. The adrenals make glucocorticoids, hormones that help increase blood sugar levels after a "crash." The more fatigued the adrenal glands are, the less capable they are of helping to stabilize blood sugar.

- Certain nutrients and botanicals help stabilize blood sugar:
    - Chromium
    - Adaptogen herbs
    - Momardica charantia
- Address adrenal (page 100) and/or thyroid (page 166) issues. These glands must be functioning well to support normal blood sugar regulation.

INDIGESTION

Indigestion usually results from eating too much food, or eating the wrong kinds of food for our particular bodies. The best treatment is prevention—eat fresh, well-cooked foods prepared and eaten in a relaxed environment. Avoid arguments while eating. Chew each bite well (some say at least 50 times). Some days, I'm lucky if I chew each bite 10 times! Eat while sitting down, preferably in a chair and not while hurtling along the freeway in your car. Remember that the digestive system works best when we are relaxed, which is when the parasympathetic nervous system is most active (see the section on "Nutrition" in Chapter 2).

- Avoid eating when you are rushed or emotionally upset. The body shunts energy and circulation away from the digestive tract during stressful periods, whether the stress is physical, mental, or emotional.
- Avoid eating excessive amounts of cold or raw food. From a Chinese medical perspective, the stomach functions best when it is warm (but not overheated). Steamed and baked foods are easiest to digest. Raw foods, as well as cold or frozen foods, tend to be very cooling and, therefore, difficult to digest. In general, the body tolerates a modest amount of raw food better in the warm summer months than during the winter.
- Avoid highly spiced, fried or greasy foods, which may overheat the digestive system and cause irritation.
- Choose water and herb teas for beverages. Avoid coffee, black tea and alcohol, all of which are heating and irritating to the digestive tract.

Botanical therapy

- Peppermint oil – Place one drop in a cup of hot water. Essential oils are very strong, so one drop really is enough.

- Ginger tea – Grate one or two tablespoons of fresh ginger into two cups of water. Bring to a boil and simmer for 10 minutes. Sip the warm tea as needed. Ginger is warming, which helps stimulate digestion.
- Chamomile and/or mint tea – Add one tablespoon of dried herb to one cup of boiling water. Allow to steep for 10 minutes, then drink.
- Pill Curing – a Chinese patent formula. Take one vial of the pellets every three or more hours as needed.

Homeopathic remedies 30c potency

- Nux vomica – classic for overeating and overdrinking. The patient tends to overwork and keep a demanding schedule, which irritates his already weak digestive system. Tendency for constipation.
- Arsenicum – burning pain in the stomach, with desire to drink small sips of water, although water may cause vomiting. Food poisoning with both diarrhea and vomiting.

When to consult a physician

- If indigestion becomes a regular occurrence (more than once or twice per week)
- If you notice changes in the bowel movements
- Black, tarry stools (may be an indication of stomach or duodenal ulcer)
- Excessive gas and bloating (may be an indication of parasite infection). This does not include gas caused by eating too many or poorly cooked beans!
- Regular or severe episodes of heartburn
- If symptoms of indigestion, bloating and burping consistently follow ingestion of fatty, greasy or rich foods (may be a symptom of gall bladder irritation)

INSECT AND OTHER BITES

In general, clean the wound with soap and water.

Botanical therapy

- Calendula succus (plant juice, preserved with a small amount of alcohol)—encourages wound healing and prevents infection. Apply after washing the bite.

- Comfrey or mullein compresses—also encourage healing. Comfrey contains allantoin, a plant constituent that increases cell division and thereby speeds wound healing. Mullein has soothing properties to ease the stinging and itching associated with insect bites. Make a compress by crushing the leaves or putting fresh leaves in the blender with a small amount of water. Spread the crushed leaves on muslin or cheese-cloth and apply to the affected area.
- Fresh potato—Cut in slices and apply to affected areas to draw out inflammation and swelling.
- Bentonite clay—reconstituted to a paste and applied to the area, this will draw out inflammation and swelling and reduce pain.

Homeopathic remedies: 30c potency

- Ledum – specific for bites and puncture wounds of all kinds, especially those that are cold and pale blue in color. Ledum is especially helpful for "dirty" bites, or animal bites that are susceptible to infection.
- Cantharis – bites with intense itching, small red bumps and vesicles
- Tarantula – for spider bites
- Apis – for bee stings or any kind of sting that causes intense, painful swelling and stinging
- Hypericum – for shooting pain
- Lachesis – for snakebite

When to consult a physician

- If the insect bite becomes infected
- If you have an allergic reaction to the insect sting, e.g., excessive swelling in the local area or difficulty breathing
- If you suspect you may have been bitten by a poisonous insect

INFLAMMATORY BOWEL DISEASE

Many people currently suffer with one or more Inflammatory Bowel Diseases—ulcerative colitis, Crohn's disease and irritable bowel syndrome. Sometimes the lines between these diseases blur; patients may have one or a combination of these inflammatory conditions.

I have included a section on optimizing digestive health because this particular system is an important cornerstone for overall health. If I cannot effectively absorb nutrients and discard waste, all of the other body systems suffer.

The better the digestive tract is performing, the better all of the other systems can function.

What causes inflammation in the bowel in the first place? Two major contributing factors are diet and stress levels.

How stress impacts your digestive tract

When the body is under stress, the adrenal glands dump epinephrine, norepinephrine and a host of other hormones into the bloodstream. These hormones are intended to prepare the body to fight or run away, the "fight or flight" response. The body shunts blood away from the digestive tract into the muscles, lungs and heart, to prepare for quick movement. In these "emergency" situations, the digestive system is not important; the immediate concerns of fighting or running are more important.

Unfortunately, the body responds the same way whether the "stressor" is a bear chasing you in the woods or an angry driver honking in rush hour traffic. The stress-related hormones are meant to help the body *move*, to respond to the "danger," whether it is perceived or real. Instead of moving, though, most of us sit still. We nod at the angry boss, or draw our shoulders up to our ears as we inch forward in rush hour traffic.

The body does not "use up" these stress related hormones until we finally *move*. Exercise is a key player in utilizing the hormones. Without movement, adrenalin continues to circulate in the body, causing a narrowing of the blood vessels that support the digestive tract. This decreased circulation means the digestive tract is functioning at sub-optimal levels. Even eating the freshest, nutrient-rich, organic produce will have little benefit if we are unable to digest the food.

Stress challenges anyone's digestive tract. If the stomach and intestines are already sensitive or weakened, the stress impacts these organs even more.

How food impacts the digestive tract

The second major factor that influences digestive function is the food we eat. We understand why poorly fed pets or farm animals sicken and die. Unfortunately, many of us think our own bodies are immune to the same laws.

The tricky part here is that what constitutes optimal food varies from person to person. I cannot offer any patient a one-size-fits-all diet. Although some foundation information is applicable to everyone, e.g., the need for essential nutrients and fatty acids in the body ("essential" means nutrients the body cannot produce, that must be ingested as food), *no one food is good for everyone.*

I recommend food testing for many patients who have chronic conditions, even if they seem unrelated to the digestive tract. Any chronic inflammatory condition, such as arthritis, eczema, asthma, sinusitis or heart disease, improves when you reduce overall inflammation in the body.

Constitutional food intolerance, ALCAT and/or allergy testing can help you to identify foods that trigger inflammation in your particular body. The following foods generally increase inflammation, whether or not they are allergens or intolerances, because of their acidifying effect on the body:

- Alcohol
- Coffee
- Refined carbohydrates (white flour, white sugar, white rice, etc.)
- Meat and animal products (eggs, dairy)

These foods are the mainstay of most people's diets in industrialized countries. The more you eat of these foods, whether you are allergic to them or not, the more inflammation you will have in the digestive tract in particular and the body in general.

For more information on the effects of food intolerances and food allergies, see page 31.

Treating inflammatory bowel disease

You can follow two primary roads in treating digestive problems and travel both of these roads at the same time: Reduce inflammation in the digestive tract and rebuild the gut.

Reducing inflammation in the gut involves removing foods and additives that generally inflame the gut and that are difficult for any digestive tract to process. Ideally, you would also identify and remove foods that specifically irritate your particular digestive tract. Refer to the section above about identifying food intolerances and food allergies, as well as foods that increase inflammation in the digestive tract.

The second, equally important road to follow is rebuilding the digestive tract. Sadly, conventional medicine has lost most, if not all information about how to restore function in the body. Classical medicines still retain a wide variety of methods to rebuild the digestive tract. This rebuilding work is the foundation of any other treatments for this part of the body. You could be taking fistfuls of pills to support digestion, but if the digestive organs are not working well, you will have little to no benefit from the medicines.

- The constitutional hydrotherapy treatment (page 55) increases blood flow in the digestive tract. Remember that increased stress triggers hormones that constrict the blood vessels that nourish the digestive tract. Diminished blood flow means reduced digestive function, including tissue repair work. Increasing blood flow encourages the digestive tract to heal. As a bonus, the constitutional hydrotherapy treatment also boosts red–and-white blood cell production and activity. I have had patients on chemotherapy who have been able to maintain their white blood cell count by doing the constitutional hydrotherapy treatment on a regular (usually daily) basis.

- Acupuncture: the National Institute of Health (NIH) and the World Health Organization (WHO) include digestive disorders among the long list of conditions that are at least 90 percent effectively treated by acupuncture. In the West, most people think of acupuncture as treating only musculoskeletal conditions. Each of the "meridians" or channels, however, connects with an internal organ. Needling points on the body directly affects internal organ function.

- Abdominal massage has been practiced for millennia as a way of relaxing the muscles that surround the digestive tract and increasing blood flow to the organs themselves. You can increase the activity of the colon by massage along its natural course: up the right side of the body, across the abdomen and down the left side. Gently massaging in this circular motion around the abdomen can relax intestinal cramps and encourage normal peristalsis, the wave-like muscles contractions that move food through the upper gastrointestinal tract and then waste through the lower digestive tract.

- Cleansing helps to remove the backlog of accumulated waste in the lower digestive tract. Most of us have an accumulation of feces and/or mucoid plaque, even if we have regular, daily bowel movements. We can safely, gently remove this accumulated waste with appropriate cleansing programs. By "appropriate" I mean staying within the body's carrying capacity—in this case, the electrolyte levels necessary to remove waste products. Electrolytes are the minerals in the body that facilitate many biochemical processes. If electrolyte levels are low, the body does not have the "hardware" necessary to remove waste products. Trying to push the body to cleanse when electrolyte levels are low will do more harm than good to the body as a whole. PLEASE check pH levels, which are a reflection of electrolyte levels, before you begin any cleanse program. See page 137 for information about how to test pH levels and how bentonite clay can aid your cleansing routine.

- Avoid cathartic herbs to clear the intestines. Many companies now offer "intestinal cleanse" programs. Most of these programs involve eating your normal diet and taking large amounts of cathartic herbs that *irritate* the intestines, thereby causing more bowel movements. In the short-term (e.g., up to four weeks), using cathartic herbs can support the intestines in removing waste. Using these herbs for extended periods of time, however, can cause overproduction of melanin in the intestines. Some studies suggest that this increase in melanin production may lead to colon cancer.

  Recently, a patient in her mid-thirties who already had a long history of digestive problems had a colonoscopy. Already, at this relatively young age, she had melanosis in the colon. She had been using cathartic herbs once or twice *a month* for several years. Even this seemingly low level use of cathartic herbs had significantly irritated her large intestine.

  Over time the intestines become habituated to the irritating effects of the cathartic herbs, just as the intestines can become habituated to pharmaceutical drugs for constipation. When the intestines are habituated, these herbs no longer trigger a bowel movement.

  Cathartic herbs for short-term use only: senna and buckthorn bark (*Cascara sagrada*).

Dietary suggestions

- Increase dietary fiber, particularly digestible fibers. Our digestive tracts thrive with a combination of digestible and indigestible fiber. "Digestible" fibers include pectin, flaxseed meal and oat bran. These fibrous foods lubricate as well as bulk the stools. Indigestible fibers, such as wheat bran and psyllium seed husks, "sweep" waste matter out of the intestines. Both digestible and indigestible fibers also reduce fat and cholesterol uptake in the gut. NOTE: If you increase fiber, you also need to increase fluid intake. If you increase fiber without drinking more *non*-caffeinated fluids, the fiber will simply bind up the stools even more.

- Increase fluids. If you are even slightly dehydrated, the body reabsorbs water across the intestines and back into general circulation. Waste products meant for removal through the intestines are also reabsorbed along with the water into the bloodstream. The more dehydrated you are, the more water is reabsorbed from the intestines. As a result, the stools become harder and move more slowly through the intestines. Increasing water intake is one the simplest and most effective ways to improve intestinal health.

- Reduce or eliminate meat and animal products (e.g., dairy and eggs). These foods are naturally high in arachadonic acid, a fatty acid that runs inflammatory pathways. The more meat and meat products you eat, the more the body produces inflammatory compounds called leukotrienes. Increased inflammation in turn triggers intestinal cramping and pain.

- For those suffering with ulcerative colitis, eliminate carrageenan, a seaweed extract used to thicken a wide variety of packaged foods. Patients with ulcerative colitis tend to have up to six times the normal levels of *Bacteroides vulgatus*. Carrageenan is a preferred food for these particular bacteria. Carrageenan does not trigger intestinal damage in people who have normal levels of *Bacteroides vulgatus*.

- Eliminate coffee, black tea and caffeinated sodas. Caffeine acts as a diuretic—e.g., you lose two-to-three cups of fluid for each cup of caffeinated drink you consume. Caffeinated beverages count *against* your overall fluid intake and will help further bind the stools. Even decaffeinated coffee and black tea have some diuretic effects. Red raspberry leaf tea is a great substitute for black tea. Naturally high in tannins, red raspberry leaf tea tastes almost exactly like black tea. I am referring here to tea from the red raspberry plant (*Rubus ideaus*), NOT black tea flavored like raspberry.

- Drink slippery elm bark tea or eat slippery elm bark lozenges. Slippery elm bark is a demulcent, meaning it soothes and lubricates the digestive tract (and the urinary tract as well). This smooth inner bark of the elm tree also has some nutritive properties. Slippery elm bark is safe for long-term use. Other demulcent herbs include marshmallow root and deglycyrrhizinated licorice (DGL).

- Supplement probiotics. These beneficial bacteria support the body in many ways. Some of these organisms produce B vitamins; others function as extensions of the immune system. When this beneficial flora is depleted in the intestines, certain immune system activities are diminished. This explains in part why you are more susceptible to new infections if you do not restore these beneficial bacteria after taking antibiotics.

Probiotics vary widely in quality. Look for sources that test microscopically to make sure that they are culturing exactly what they say on the label. These bacteria easily mutate, so some of the supplements on the shelf contain distant cousins of the organisms listed on the label. Ideally, the probiotics would include several different organisms, not just acidophilus. Finally, fructo-oligosaccharides (FOS) are the preferred food of the healthy intestinal flora. Supplements that include FOS give the probiotics an extra boost in re-establishing themselves in the gut.

Take one teaspoon of flaxseed oil, one-to-two times per day. Flaxseed oil is rich in Omega-3 essential fatty acids and helps to run the anti-inflammatory pathways in the body. Flaxseed oil must be refrigerated and should never be heated or cooked. Light, air and heat quickly oxidize flaxseed oil. NOTE: You must take flaxseed oil, or any supplemental oil, with a protein in order for the oil to be absorbed across the intestines. The protein polarizes the fat molecule so that it can be absorbed across the intestinal barrier. "Protein" does not necessarily mean meat. You can add flaxseed oil to cooked oatmeal, or a salad that includes nuts or whole grains.

INSOMNIA

Most Western treatments for insomnia focus on the nervous system. Conventional over-the-counter and pharmaceutical medications simply "knock out" the nervous system. Western botanical medicine focuses on "nervines," herbs that both nourish and calm the nervous system. None of the prescription medications "nourish" the nerves; in fact, most of them disrupt the normal sleep "architecture," the brain wave patterns that fluctuate during a restful night's sleep.

Chinese medicine approaches insomnia from a completely different direction. Insomnia results from an increase of heat in the heart. This does NOT mean that if you stuck a thermometer in the heart, it would literally register a hotter temperature. The Chinese are referring to a more subtle, internal change. Normally, the spirit, or *shen,* in the body rests in the heart when we go to sleep. If the heart is heated or agitated, the heart does not have a quiet place to rest and we have difficulty falling asleep and/or staying asleep. Instead of knocking out the nervous system, Chinese herbalists prescribe medicinals that nourish and cool the heart. Usually, these herbs are taken throughout the day instead of just at bedtime.

James Maas, Ph.D., a sleep researcher and author of several books and television documentaries, offers sound advice about improving sleep. Most humans, according to Maas' research, need nine-to-10 hours of sleep to function normally. A century ago most people in this culture slept nine-to-10 hours. Now, if you mention to someone that you regularly sleep more than eight hours, they would likely call you "lazy"! In truth, most of us need this amount of sleep. A few immortals truly can function well on four-to-five hours of sleep; some need closer to 12. The average for humans is nine-to-10 hours.

If we are sleep-deprived, the two major systems in the body that suffer are the nervous and the immune systems. Concentration and memory are the first mental functions to suffer. Research at the Henry Ford Sleep Clinic revealed that increasing sleep by one hour per day increases concentration by 25 percent! If we are sleep-deprived, several immune markers drop, leaving us more susceptible to colds, the flu and other infections.

Many people assume they have slept enough because they wake at a certain hour in the morning. Waking at a particular time usually has more to do with the *body clock* than with the body actually having enough rest. Our body clocks are conditioned by our daily schedule. If we have to get up for work or school at a certain time each day, eventually the body clock is set to wake at that time. Trying to shift the body clock can lead to a whole range of problems, which we see twice a year when we go off or on Daylight Savings Time.

The point here is that the body's "natural" waking time does not necessarily mean that the body is fully rested. If you have a drop in energy or concentration during the day, you are not getting enough sleep.

Good sleep hygiene is the foundation for improving your sleep patterns. Dr. Maas suggests keeping the same waking time, seven days a week, and then gradually moving back your bedtime. If you go to sleep at 11 p.m. and wake at 5:30 a.m., for example, keep the same waking time each day and gradually move back your bedtime by 15 minutes each week. The first week, go to bed at 10:45 p.m. The next week go to sleep at 10:30 p.m. Continue to gradually move your bedtime earlier and earlier until you reach a point that you have even concentration and energy throughout your day.

Dr. Maas advises against sleeping in on the weekends (something I'm definitely guilty of). Sleeping later in the morning means we usually are up later at night. Sunday night, feeling well rested, I might stay up an hour later. The next morning, the alarm rings at the usual, early time and I am once again scrambling to catch up with sleep. Instead of sleeping in to repay our sleep deficit, Dr. Maas recommends keeping a consistent sleep pattern, seven days a week.

As mentioned earlier, pharmaceutical drugs disrupt our normal brain wave patterns during sleep. Usually, we enter deep sleep for the first two-to-three hours and then brainwave patterns shift to rapid eye movement (REM) sleep for a few minutes. As the sleep cycle progresses, we spend more and more time in REM cycle sleep, until by 6.5 hours we are almost exclusively in REM sleep.

During REM sleep, short-term memory moves to long-term memory and a whole range of other restorative processes in the body take place. Most of us are getting up precisely when the body is entering the most restorative portion of the sleep cycle. One sleep study explored the effect of disrupting the sleep cycle every time participants moved into REM sleep. Within a few days, all of the study participants became psychotic. The study had to be halted. REM is an extremely important part of the sleep cycle and one that most of us are short-changing because of our sleep habits.

If we are not sleeping enough, over time we develop a sleep deficit. Sleeping well for one night, or even one week, won't repay that deficit. Maas suggests increasing sleep for at least six-to-eight weeks to refill the deficit. In my experience, having become severely sleep-deprived several times in my life, I needed months, not weeks, to repay the lack of sleep.

Sleep is an absolute foundation for health, as important as breathing or drinking water. All of the fancy supplements in the world cannot make up for a lack of sleep. Consider good sleep an absolute must for good health.

Many health factors can contribute to insomnia. This section will address the majority of the causes, but certainly not all. If you have followed these suggestions for six months and have no improvement in your sleep patterns, discuss your situation with your family physician to consider other options.

- Establish regular sleep habits. Create a consistent waking time and a regular bedtime.
- Slow down the hour before going to bed. I have patients who are, figuratively and sometimes, literally, running right up to the time they go to bed. The body has difficulty slowing down and settling into sleep if you are engaged in activities right up to the time of trying to go to sleep.
- Choose slower, more relaxing activities the hour before sleep. You might finish writing a letter, take frozen food out of the freezer to thaw for tomorrow's dinner, brush your teeth, etc. This is an excellent time to stretch, do a bit of yoga, or for some, practice qigong. I say "for some" because qigong practice can either soothe and relax someone, preparing her for sleep, or deeply energize the body. If you are someone for whom yoga and/or qigong is deeply energizing, schedule your practice sessions in the morning.
- Eliminate caffeine. If you are a regular coffee drinker, this one suggestion, more than any other, can dramatically improve your sleep. Even

if you drink one cup of coffee in the morning, that dose of caffeine can alter sleep cycles. If you are a regular coffee drinker, gradually reduce your coffee intake to avoid withdrawal headaches. By "gradual," I mean reduce your coffee intake by half a cup per week. This may take longer if you are a major coffee drinker, but you are likely to be successful with gradual reduction. One of the best coffee substitutes I have found is Teeccino®. This brewed coffee replacement can be substituted gradually for coffee. Remember that the taste will never be exactly the same. You'll have to learn to like Teeccino for itself. Some people enjoy a cup of hot water instead of the coffee, once the weaning process is complete. You'll find your own way.

- Exercise regularly. Aerobic exercise at least four days a week can make a big difference in your sleep. Most of us live very stressful lives. Under stress, we produce more cortisol and other adrenal hormones. These hormones are meant to increase heart and breathing rates and shunt the blood away from the internal organs to the muscles, preparing us to fight or run away. The only way we "use up" these stress related hormones is to MOVE! Most of us, though, have to stay at our desk, or continue to care for the children, after a major stress. We don't get up and move. Instead, the stress-related hormones continue to surge in our bloodstream for days or weeks at a time. These hormones can disrupt our ability to relax and sleep. Exercise can "use up" the hormones and improve our sleep patterns.

- Use ear plugs. Unless you have young children or an elderly parent you must attend to, ear plugs can eliminate much of the uncontrollable noise that can disrupt sleep patterns.

- Eliminate artificial light exposure. Streetlights and lights left on in the house can disrupt the pineal gland. This gland plays an important role in regulating the sleep cycle. If necessary, wear an eye mask to eliminate external light exposure.

- Meditate before going to sleep. This relaxes the body and the mind, preparing both for relaxation and sleep.

- My favorite sleep aide is a guided relaxation that is over 4,000 years old. "Four Route Relaxation" is an ancient lying-down relaxation form of qigong (see Chapter 2 for an introduction to qigong). You can play the CD as you fall asleep. You do not need to try to stay awake as you listen; some part of the mind is listening even while you are asleep. NOTE: Because this particular relaxation exercise involves discharging stale or stagnant energy from the body, *make sure that no pets or chil-*

dren are in the room when you are doing this relaxation exercise. Pets and children are especially vulnerable to absorbing other people's discharged energies, because their own energetic bodies are not as well developed as an adult human. To order a copy of the CD, visit http://drjudithboice.3dcartstores.com/Relaxation-CD_p_78.html

- The first, gentlest intervention is to drink a cup of nervine tea at bedtime. The nervines are a class of herbs that both calm and nourish the nervous system. Brew a heaping teaspoon of the dried herb in a cup of boiling water. Allow to steep for 10 minutes and then drink. You can maximize the volatile oils in the tea by placing a small plate on top of the cup to trap the steam.

  - Chamomile (*Matricaria rescutita*) – My current favorite is Traditional Medicinals Chamomile with Lavender tea, already in tea bags. High in calcium, chamomile gently soothes the nervous system and helps prepare for sleep.

  - Skullcap (*Scutellaria lateriflora*) – Also high in calcium, this herb calms and nourishes the nervous system. Skullcap is beneficial for anxiety, restless sleep, nervous exhaustion and nervous system weakness after a long illness.

  - Valerian (*Valeriana officinalis*) – a much stronger nervine. Beloved by cats, this herbs smells like dirty socks to me. Others love its pungent taste. Too much valerian can have opposite effects, actually stimulating the nervous system rather than soothing it.

  - Passion flower (*Passiflora incarnata*) – This herb soothes muscle spasms, heart palpitations and nervousness, all of which can contribute to sleep disturbances.

  - Hops (*Humulus lupulus*) – addresses irritable digestive tract and nervous system (indigestion and sleeplessness). Hops is very specific for soothing nervousness with muscle twitching. This muscle relaxing property also makes hops a wonderful aide for menstrual cramping.

  - Kava kava (*Piper methysticum*) – this nervine herb calms the nervous system without sedating the mind. Kava relieves anxiety and stress, insomnia and muscle tension. Caution: Long-term, high dose use of Kava can cause dry, pigmented, scaly skin, particularly on the palms of the hands, soles of the feet, back and shins. This condition, called "kava-ism," is more common in the South Pacific where people drink Kava much like North Americans drink coffee. The rash disappears when someone stops drinking Kava kava tea.

- Chinese herbs: the Chinese herbs have a radically different way of supporting sleep. Instead of knocking out the nervous system, the Chinese herbalist aims to nourish and "cool" the heart. My favorite formula for "Heart *yin* deficiency" (heart heat generated by a lack of the nourishing, cooling aspects of the body) is Ardisia 16, made by Seven Forests (Institute for Traditional Medicine in Portland, Oregon). Most health food stores do not carry Chinese medicinals, in large part because very few, if any, people working in health food stores are trained in Chinese medicine. The Chinese have a much more highly developed system of creating herbal formulas than we do in the West (see the introduction to Chinese herbal medicine). Ideally, you would work with a Chinese herbalist to create the most appropriate formula for your particular situation.

- Flower essences:
  - Rescue Remedy®: See information in the Flower Essence section in Chapter 2.
  - Chamomile: Calms emotional upset, especially emotions held in the stomach. I used this with my boys when they were small. This is a gentle, effective way to help children "wind down" for sleep. Although the flower essences did not "knock out" the boys, they definitely were calmer as they approached sleep.
  - Aspen: fear of the unknown, the dark; hypersensitive to unseen forces, real or imagined
  - Black-Eyed Susan: difficulty sleeping that is related to troubling thoughts that are repressed or only dimly conscious; subconscious is trying to relieve itself of toxic material
  - Chaparral: cathartic dreams that trouble the psyche and disrupt sleep
  - Dill: insomnia due to nervous or sensory overwhelm
  - Lavender: "wired" nervous system, especially from extreme mental or spiritual pursuits
  - Mugwort: overactive dreams disturb sleep
  - Red chestnut: sleep disrupted by excessive worry or over-concern for others
  - Saint John's Wort: disturbing dreams; fears or psychic stress of any kind

- White Chestnut: repetitive, obsessive thoughts disrupt sleep; unable to quiet the mind

Other supplements that support sleep include:

- Melatonin: This hormone produced by the pineal gland helps set the "body clock" that regulates sleeping and waking cycles. Melatonin has a normal "diurnal rhythm," meaning that levels rise and fall in a regular pattern throughout a 24-hour cycle. Normally, melatonin peaks between midnight and 2 a.m. If you take melatonin during or shortly before these hours, you will delay the normal peak and, thus, the normal drop in levels. Instead of melatonin dropping to a low level by 9 a.m., the late-night dose ensures that melatonin levels are still riding high in the early morning, thus causing a "hangover" effect. Ideally, you would take a maximum of 3 mg of melatonin (more than that should be taken under a doctor's supervision) by 8:30 or 9 p.m. This dosing schedule will support the body's normal melatonin pattern.
- 5-HTP: A precursor to L-tryptophan, 5-HTP became available after L-tryptophan was taken off the market (because of a manufacturing error in a production plant in Japan, NOT because of any safety concerns about L-tryptophan itself). 5-HTP is a precursor to serotonin, which profoundly effects sleep cycle, depression, appestat (appetite control) and many other functions in the body. For insomnia, take 100-to-300 mg of 5-HTP, 30-to-45 minutes before bedtime. Start with the lower dose for at least three days before increasing the dosage.
- Calcium and magnesium: These two minerals are closely paired cousins in their effect on relaxing muscles and supporting heart function. These nutrients can be very helpful in addressing restless leg syndrome, another common cause of poor sleep. Ideally, these minerals are always taken together. Because they are both absorbed across the intestine in a similar way, a large dose of one will artificially drive down the absorption of the other. Although the exact correct ratio of calcium to magnesium has not been established (and the truth is that ratio likely varies slightly from person to person), always take at least half as much magnesium as calcium. If you take 500 mg of calcium, for example, take *at least* 250 mg of magnesium. Taking too much calcium and magnesium can soften or loosen the stools. If you have loose stools, reduce the dosage and then see if you can gradually increase the amount you are taking.

A final note about sleep: if you are enduring a prolonged period of insomnia, I would encourage you to learn to relax in bed, even if you are not sleeping. Some patients play the Four Route relaxation tape again, so that they are at least gaining the benefits of relaxation, even if they are not sleeping. Some people meditate during these hours and gain the benefits of mental relaxation, even when the body is not fully resting. An interesting note: Many meditators on extended retreats discover they do not need as much sleep. The prolonged periods in deep, relaxed mental concentration seem to fill a similar function as sleep.

MOTION SICKNESS

General recommendations

- Relaxation exercises, before and during travel. Move through the body from head to foot, noting and releasing any areas of muscle tension. Take up to 10 deep breaths and allow your body to grow heavy and relaxed.
- Drink ginger tea. Grate one or two tablespoons of fresh ginger into a saucepan with two cups of water. Bring to a boil and then simmer for 10 minutes. Drink one-half cup of ginger tea every half hour, or as needed for stomach upset.
- Mint and chamomile teas also soothe the stomach. Steep one tablespoon dried herb in a cup of boiling water for 10 minutes. Drink as needed.
- Apply pressure to Pericardium 6 (PC6), an acupuncture point associated with calming the digestive tract and reducing nausea. You can wear a bracelet that applies pressure on this point. Sea Band™ makes these bands in adult and children's sizes.

Homeopathic remedies 30c potency

Take the remedy one hour before travel, then as needed once travel begins.
- Borax – for motion sickness during air travel. Symptoms worsen with downward motion.
- Rhus tox – nausea and vomiting with complete loss of appetite. Giddiness on attempting to rise. Severe frontal headache. Unquenchable thirst.
- Cocculus – for car sickness. Also for morning sickness in pregnancy. Person cannot stand the sight or smell of food. Hollow, empty feeling.

When to consult a physician

- If the above remedies do not alleviate motion sickness.
- If you have difficulties with balance that are exacerbated by travel. You may have an inner-ear problem that needs further treatment.

PHYSICAL TRAUMA

Most trauma is caused by stretching tissues beyond their capacity. Overstretching connective tissues (muscle, blood vessels, tendons, bones) leads to tissue damage, pain and swelling. Swelling may serve as a natural splint, to protect and immobilize the traumatized area. Unfortunately, swelling may also lead to a dangerous decrease in circulation.

The treatments listed below apply to most physical injuries. Please see other sections of this chapter for information on specific conditions (bruising, burns, etc.).

- Give homeopathic Arnica as soon as possible after the injury. Arnica is specific for trauma, bruising, head injury and soft-tissue injury and can also slow bleeding and treat shock. Often someone needing Arnica will deny that she is injured. Imagine a construction worker falling two stories, landing hard, getting up and saying she is fine— she needs Arnica!
- Continue giving Arnica as needed for three-to-four days, or longer if you have a major injury. You may repeat the remedy as often as every 30 minutes immediately after the injury. Remember, homeopathic remedies act according to the frequency of dosage, not the amount.
- For the first 24 hours, use cold applications on the affected area. Leave the cold pack on for a maximum of ten minutes at a time. Take a break for a few minutes; then, reapply the cold pack. There is some controversy here: One school of thought says cold applications are best because they reduce circulation and, therefore, swelling, in the local area; another school of thought argues that cold applications cause "stagnation" (as defined in Chinese medicine) by slowing the circulation. A compromise approach involves alternating hot and cold applications to increase circulation and decrease stagnation.
- After 24 hours, use alternating hot and cold applications—five minutes of hot, followed by one minute of cold. Continue for at least three cycles of alternating hot and cold applications. Always end with a cold application.

Other Homeopathic remedies: 30c potency

- Ledum – bruised area that is cold and blue. Follows Arnica well, after three or four days.
- Ruta – injury to periosteum (surface of the bone). Area is red; condition worsens with motion. Also for injuries to ligaments and tendons.
- Rhus tox – sore, painful joints that improve with warmth and motion (painful when first moved, better with continued movement).
- Hypericum – for injury to areas dense with nerve tissue (eyes, hands, genitals). Sharp, nerve-like pain.

Botanical remedies

- Arnica oil – apply to the affected area every three-to-four hours. Because Arnica is a counter-irritant (increasing circulation in an area by causing mild irritation) it should not be used on broken skin. CAUTION: for external use only. Do not take botanical Arnica internally. Use on unbroken skin only.
- Hypericum oil – causes blood-vessel dilation; warming to injured area, soothing to nerves. CAUTION: for external use only.
- Symphytum (comfrey) oil or salve – stimulates cell production and tissue healing. Apply externally, or take as tea internally. Comfrey tea is especially healing for bone breaks. CAUTION: for skin injuries (cuts and abrasions), apply comfrey only after scab formation. Applying comfrey to a deep, open wound can cause the wound to close too quickly, trapping anaerobic bacteria in the wound and possibly causing a serious infection.
- Any plant with chlorophyll will stimulate healing. Plantain is exceptionally soothing to the skin. Crush the leaves and apply to cuts and abrasions, especially if you are outdoors and have no other first-aid supplies with you. Plantain is called "nature's Band-Aid."

Acupressure: Deeply massage points on the limb opposite the injured area, or the "opposite-opposite" limb. For a left ankle injury, for example, massage the right ankle and/or the right wrist. Massaging points on the opposite or opposite-opposite joint will increase circulation in the injured area.

When to consult a physician

- If the patient shows signs of shock (see the section on "Shock," below)
- If the injury involves blood loss (more than minor oozing from a cut)

- If you cannot voluntarily move the injured area
- If you can see bone protruding through the skin
- If you begin to see red streaks developing above an injury, moving up the arm or leg—a sign of internal infection
- If pain and swelling persist for more than three-to-four days after injury.

POISON IVY AND POISON OAK

General recommendations

- Learn to identify these plants and keep a respectful distance away from them.
- Wash with soap and water. The rash and irritation associated with poison oak and ivy are caused by oil in the plant's leaves and stems. Washing with soap emulsifies and removes oils, decreasing and sometimes completely removing the irritant.
- Remove the irritant with drawing agents. Moisten bentonite clay with enough water to form a smooth paste. Add one or two drops of peppermint oil. The clay will absorb oils and oozing discharge from poison ivy rashes. A very small amount of peppermint oil will decrease itching. If you do not have clay, apply a fresh slice of potato to the area. (Potato also acts as a drawing agent.)
- Avoid touching or brushing the affected area. You may spread the irritant oil accidentally by scratching the rash and then touching another body part. This is usually how poison ivy spreads to the eyes and face. If you tend to scratch in your sleep, wear cotton gloves. Wash your hands often during the day.

Homeopathic remedies: 30c potency

- Rhus toxicodendron – for itchy, red vesicles. The area feels better with hot-water applications and motion.
- Rhus lobatum – made from poison oak, which is more common on the West Coast. Some people respond better to this remedy than to Rhus tox, which is made from poison ivy.
- If you are extremely sensitive to poison ivy or oak and must work in or near it (e.g., clearing poison ivy in your yard), take one 30c dose of Rhus tox before beginning work. This prophylactic dose can reduce and sometimes prevent a rash.

When to consult a physician

- If the rash continues to spread despite treatment
- If the rash persists for more than seven days
- If the area becomes infected

SHOCK

When someone goes into shock, the body suspends all but the most vital functions. If shock goes untreated, even those vital functions may shut down. Symptoms of shock include:

- confusion
- very slow or very fast pulse
- very slow or very fast breathing
- trembling or weakness of the arms and legs
- cool, moist skin
- enlarged pupils
- pale or bluish fingernails, lips, skin

Treatments for shock

Call 911. Most shock is caused by major trauma and requires immediate medical attention. The following suggestions are meant to support the patient until emergency medical care arrives.

- Keep the patient lying down.
- Address the cause of the shock: Remove any live electrical source (if you can do so without endangering yourself); stanch bleeding; remove causes of severe pain; use First-Aid procedures to restore breathing.
- Keep the patient warm. Cover him or her with a blanket and elevate the feet.
- Give "Rescue Remedy™," a blend of Bach flowers available at most health-food stores. Give three or four drops under the tongue every fifteen minutes, or as necessary once recovery begins.

Homeopathic remedies: 30c potency

Give every 15-to-50 minutes until improvement is noted.

- Aconite – fear, fright, anxiety. Sudden, violent onset. Numbness. Vomiting from fear. Face is deathly pale when patient sits up. Fear of death.

- Carbo veg – icy coldness. Stagnant blood. "Air hunger" (can't catch breath). Wants windows open; wants to be fanned; wants cold drinks during chills.
- Gelsemium – dull, droopy, drowsy, dazed. Dilated pupils. No thirst. Heat stroke. Heavy, drooping eyelids.
- Arnica – especially after head injury. Denies need for help ("I'm fine. Just leave me alone.").

When to consult a physician

- Always consult a physician for illnesses and injuries involving shock.
- If the patient has minor injuries (e.g., a scraped leg or arm) and does not respond to the above treatment within 10-to-15 minutes.

SUNBURN

Fair-skinned people always have been susceptible to sunburn. Now, with the increasing emissions of hydrocarbons and fluorocarbons and subsequent destruction of the ozone layer, even dark-skinned people are at risk. The long-term effects of excessive sun exposure include skin cancer. One severe sunburn during a lifetime can increase the risk of multiple myeloma, i.e., bone cancer.

The best treatment is preventive:

- Stay out of the sun during the middle of the day (11 a.m. to 3 p.m.), when the sun's rays are strongest.
- Wear hats that screen the face, especially the nose. Wear light clothing that covers the arms and legs.
- Apply sunscreen to areas of the skin that are not covered by clothing. Sunscreen increases the number of minutes the skin can withstand burning rays by the factor noted on the product. For example, a fair-skinned person without protection might normally stay in the sun for 10 minutes before noticing signs of burning. If that person uses a Sun Protection Factor (SPF) 15 sunscreen, he or she could stay in the sun for 10 x 15 minutes, or 150 minutes (i.e., 2.5 hours). Reapplying the sunscreen after 150 minutes will not increase the length of protection. Washing off the sunscreen will reduce the effective time.

If you are unable to avoid overexposure, use the following treatments:

- Apply cool water as soon as possible. Take frequent cool showers (e.g., two minutes in the shower, every one or two hours). Pat dry; do not rub the skin. If the burn is localized, apply cold wet washcloths, changing the cloth as it warms.

- Apply aloe vera gel every three-to-four hours.
- Avoid applications of oil-based products or butter. Oils and fats increase the burn, just as throwing grease on a fire will feed the flames.
- Drink plenty of fluids. Often the body becomes dehydrated, especially if the burn covers a large area of the body.

Homeopathic remedies, 30c potency

- Hypericum – for first-degree sunburn (no blistering)
- Cantharis – especially if blistering is present (second-degree burn)
- Causticum – second- and third-degree burns (blistering and/or charring)

When to consult a physician

- If a second-degree burn (i.e., with blistering) covers more than 10 percent of the skin surface.
- If the patient shows signs of:

  - heat stroke – collapse in the heat with hot, dry skin. Other symptoms include a rapid, strong pulse and high body temperature (105°F or higher). Heat stroke is a very serious condition requiring immediate medical attention.
  - heat exhaustion – collapse in the heat with moist, clammy skin. Other symptoms include profuse perspiration, weakness, nausea, dizziness, headaches and possibly cramps. Heat exhaustion is a serious condition, although not as life-threatening as heat stroke.

TEETH AND DENTAL CARE

Our teeth, the foundation of our digestive tract, enable us to grind food into smaller pieces and prepare food for the digestive process. In the mouth, saliva rich with amylase, an enzyme that begins carbohydrate digestion, mixes with the food. Already the digestive process has begun, even before we swallow food.

The teeth reflect the health of our bone as well as the digestive tract. Gum recession may be one of the first signals that bone density has diminished and more testing and treatment is necessary.

Frequent cavities also may signal changes in calcification in the body. I never had cavities until after delivering and then nursing twins. The old adage of losing a tooth for each child delivered was partially true for me. The pH changes in the mouth during pregnancy and nursing can also trigger increased cavity formation.

Poor dental hygiene encourages the growth of certain bacteria in the mouth, some of which are damaging for other tissues in the body, including the heart and kidney.

The dental hygiene habits we develop as children can carry us through a lifetime. If we establish poor habits early, we may have more difficulty later correcting them. Start your children with good dental habits and take the opportunity to improve your own. You will be rewarded with improved overall health.

Foods that support dental health

Eating naturally crunchy foods can help "clean" teeth. Apples, for example, naturally scour plaque and other debris from the teeth. Sticky, gooey candies stick to the teeth and encourage tooth decay. Sugar is acidic and begins to eat away the enamel surface of the teeth. Bacteria trapped between the teeth and at the gum line feed on sugar and speed the process of enamel deterioration.

Usually, in the earliest phase of tooth decay, the tooth is sensitive to cold; later the tooth is sensitive to heat and cold and painful as the decay penetrates the enamel coating and begins to destroy the inner pulp. Sugary foods, particularly those left in contact with teeth for extended periods of time, encourage tooth decay. Leaving young children to fall asleep with a bottle, for example, leaves the naturally sugary milk in contact with the teeth all night long, thereby speeding tooth decay.

Tooth brushing and flossing

Tooth brushing helps to remove the leftover debris of food and some plaque build up from the teeth. Check with your dental hygienist about the best brushing methods for your teeth. Generally small circular motions, rather than scrubbing back and forth, are best for cleaning the surface of the teeth. Develop your own technique, e.g., a consistent pattern, to ensure that you clean every surface of the teeth—front, back and grinding surface. Make a habit of brushing for at least a minute, after each major meal.

Flossing helps remove food, plaque accumulation and bacterial colonies from between the teeth. Flossing can also benefit the gums. Although flossing may not completely remove plaque and bacteria, it can *disrupt* the colonies enough to thwart their growth.

Teach your children to brush and floss their teeth when they are young. You can buy rubber finger caps to massage and clean your infant's gums, which helps to prevent bacteria formation in an infant's mouth. This regular cleaning also helps prepare your baby for later dental care.

Thankfully, you can find many fun, kid-friendly toothbrushes to entice children to brush. Make your own toothpaste or dentifrice with your kids (see "recipes" below) so that they are more interested in regular brushing. Find a colorful timer they can set to remind them to brush for a full minute.

Flossing may be more exciting with the specially designed flossers. I personally don't like the added environmental waste of the disposable plastic "heads" but I am willing to tolerate the waste short-term if the boys are willing to use them for flossing.

Tongue brushing and scraping

As your children learn to brush their teeth, make sure they also brush their tongue and inner cheeks. The ancient Ayurvedic tradition of scraping the tongue is finding a foothold in American dentistry. Scraping or brushing the tongue significantly reduces bacteria in the mouth. Many toothbrushes now have a "nubby" surface on the back of the brush that can be used to brush the tongue and inner cheek areas. You can also buy a tongue scraper from your local health food store or your dentist, if she is familiar with this dental research.

Fluoride treatments and cavity prevention

When I was a kid, fluoride was the darling of the dental world. Fluoride was known to support strong tooth development and routinely was added to municipal water supplies. Unfortunately, fluoride, or *aluminum* fluoride, is also a known toxin. Adding fluoride to the municipal water supplies exposed people to aluminum who did not *need* to be. The most important time for fluoride exposure is during tooth development in our childhood years. Exposure after age 12 is not particularly beneficial and in fact may be detrimental to our health.

Instead of exposing the entire population to aluminum fluoride, the best strategy is to have concentrated fluoride treatments that deliver a high dose of fluoride in a short period of time. Dentists have special gels and other treatments to expose teeth to fluoride in a clinical setting.

Avoid toothpastes that deliver fluoride on a daily basis. The toothpaste tubes warn children NOT to swallow the paste. Most kids, however, inadvertently swallow some toothpaste. No one can completely rinse the paste from their mouth. Over time, we have ongoing, small exposures to aluminum fluoride if we are regularly using fluoride-enriched toothpaste.

Xylitol and cavity prevention

More recent research has demonstrated that xylitol, a naturally occurring sugar, inhibits *Mutans streptococci* bacteria, which is known to cause tooth decay. Xylitol also promotes re-mineralization of tooth enamel. Xylitol does NOT have the toxic side effects associated with aluminum fluoride. Although studies in the 1970's demonstrated that xylitol was at least as effective as fluoride in preventing tooth decay, fluoride continues to be the recommended choice for cavity prevention.

Xylitol is a natural sugar found in many fruits and vegetables. The FDA has approved xylitol as a dietary sweetener. Xylitol has little effect on blood sugar levels and has 40 percent fewer calories than sucrose (cane sugar).

Ideally, you would have several small "doses" of xylitol throughout the day, especially immediately after meals. An enjoyable way of delivering xylitol to the teeth is chewing xylitol sweetened gum (Xylichew and other brands.) These chewing gums actually help support tooth and mouth health, instead of damaging the teeth as conventionally sweetened chewing gums do. I am happy to offer my kids the xylitol- sweetened gum to chew.

Aim for a total of 6-to-10 grams of xylitol spread over three-to-five "doses" per day. Most xylitol-sweetened chewing gums contain 1.5 grams of xylitol per piece, so chewing one-to-two pieces of gum after each meal would reach the minimum recommended dose of xylitol for cavity prevention.

Xylitol is safe for children, pregnant women and nursing mothers. Eating too much xylitol can cause gas and diarrhea.

For those who choose to use xylitol as a general sweetener, e.g., in baking and cooking, please note that the intestines may need time to adjust to this different type of sugar. Although a natural sugar derived from plants, xylitol usually is present only in small quantities in the plant. Our digestive tract is not used to breaking down and absorbing large quantities of this particular naturally-occurring sugar. You may experience a lot of gas until the digestive tract adjusts to digesting xylitol. If your digestive tract reacts to xylitol, start with small amounts and gradually increase over time.

Limiting sweets helps support overall health by stabilizing blood sugar and reducing acid formation in the body. The more simple carbohydrates, animal products, caffeine and alcohol you consume, the more acidic your body becomes. The more acidic the body, the greater the tooth decay in the mouth. Limiting sugar supports dental hygiene as well as overall health.

Most toothpaste contains sodium laurel and/or laureth sulphate, or SLS. Animal research has demonstrated that SLS is a carcinogen; these studies have not been repeated on humans. Sodium laurel sulphate and sodium laureth sulphate are foaming agents considered safe by the FDA, as long as you do not have "repeated exposures" on a daily basis. Most of us, however, have numerous exposures on a daily basis because we use multiple products containing SLS including dishwashing liquid, laundry soap, bar or liquid soap, shampoo and toothpaste.

Over time I have discovered products that do not contain SLS. The main toothpastes I have found are Homeodent, made by Boiron; and Homeofresh by Unda/Seroyal. Homeofresh also contains xylitol, to help prevent cavities. Other personal care and home care products that do NOT contain SLS include Avalon (shampoo, conditioner, lotions); and Earth Friendly (dishwashing liquid and other house cleaning products).

Gum recession

After cavity prevention, the next major concern for dental care as we age is gum recession. As bone density diminishes, the gums tend to recede, exposing the roots of the teeth that do not have a protective enamel coating. Gum recession exposes these roots, making them more prone to decay. Most dentists now have technology to assess gum recession. If you have pockets of recessed tissue, bacteria love to populate those pockets and cause infection.

These infected pockets are called "periodontal disease" and usually are surgically removed. The gum surgery can be very painful and inconvenient.

You can help minimize the development of these bacteria-rich pockets by flossing regularly and using dental probes to gently stimulate the area around the tooth root. Most of these tools look like miniature bottle brushes. Used gently, they help scour away accumulated plaque and bacteria.

You can also help reduce bacterial formation by using a drop or two of tea tree essential oil on your tooth brush or dental probe. Tea tree essential oil inhibits bacteria, viruses and fungi growth. Ideally you would have at least two essential oils that you use and rotate every one to two weeks. Remember that ongoing exposure to any one essential oil on a daily basis can increase the possibility of becoming sensitive to that particular essential oil and to the entire class of essential oils.

Treatment recommendations

- Make your own toothpaste. This can be especially fun for kids and may increase their interest in tooth brushing. This is also a way to avoid exposure to fluoride and SLS. Combine ½ cup of baking soda with 1 teaspoon of xylitol. Add enough vegetable glycerin to make a smooth paste. Add 4-to-5 drops of essential oil to flavor the paste. Store the paste in a glass jar with a tightly fitting lid. Usually the paste will last for a month. Make small quantities regularly.

- You can make a dry dentifrice by adding a few drops of essential oil to a mixture of baking soda and xylitol. Place a small amount of the powder in the palm of your hand, wet the toothbrush and dip the toothbrush into the powder. This powder mixture travels well.

- Suggested essential oils to reduce bacterial overgrowth: tea tree, myrrh, cinnamon.

- Supplement with alfalfa tablets to strengthen teeth. Alfalfa is an extraordinary plant that sends roots three-to-four *feet* into the ground to scavenge for nutrient-rich minerals in the soil. Remember that we absorb minerals more easily from a plant than an animal base. Twenty years ago, after my mother's dentist recommended surgery to correct her receding gums, I suggested she take alfalfa tablets at every meal. At her next dental check up, the dentist did not mention gum surgery and has not recommended it since. Take two-to-four alfalfa tablets at each meal. Caution: Avoid alfalfa tablets if you have a known inhalant allergy ("hay" fever) to alfalfa.

- Brush your teeth for at least one minute, three times a day, after each major meal.

- Choose naturally crunchy fruits and vegetables for snack, rather than sticky, gooey, sugary treats.

Treatment suggestions for gum recession and/or periodontal disease

- After age 40, or even earlier if you show signs of gum recession, use a dental probe to clean the gum line, at least two or three times a week. If you develop bacterial pockets, you will need to clean with the dental probe on a daily basis. Add a drop of essential oil (see those listed above) to further reduce bacterial formation.

- Pack the gums with a mixture of hydrogen peroxide and baking soda; work the gum line with a stimulator, then rinse the mouth with warm water.

- Create an herbal mouth rinse that contains one or more of the following botanicals. Wise Woman Herbals (www.wisewomanherbals.com) offers this as an herbal blend called "Herbal Mouth Rinse":

  - Oregon grape root (*Mahonia species*)
  - Calendula (*Calendula officinalis*)
  - Comfrey (*Symphytum officinalis*)
  - Myrrh (*Commiphora mol mol*)
  - Witch Hazel (*Hamamelis virginiana*)
  - Wild indigo (*Baptisia tinctoria*)
  - Prickly ash (*Zanthoxylum americana*)
  - Blood root (*Sanguinaria canadensis*)
  - Cedar essential oil (*Thuja occidentalis*)
  - Tea tree essential oil (*Melaleuca alternifolia*)

- Gum recession may be a sign of bone loss in the rest of the body. If you have gum recession, talk to your family doctor about having a bone mineral density scan to check overall bone density. The current "gold standard" for bone density testing is the DEXA scan (Dual Energy X-ray Absorptiometry). The heel scans, usually done in a basin of water, are rough screens. The DEXA will give much more accurate information.

Flower Essences for dental care

- To reduce the trauma of dental work, take a dose of Rescue Remedy™ flower essence (four drops under the tongue) before and after dental work. If you are frightened of going to the dentist, take Rescue Remedy™ even for dental cleanings.

Homeopathic remedies for dental care

- *Arnica 30c* For dental surgeries (filling cavities, root canals, etc), take a dose of homeopathic Arnica 30c before the dental work, immediately after and then every one-to-three hours as needed for pain and swelling. After wisdom teeth extraction or other major surgeries, you likely will need a liquid preparation of the remedy rather than the usual sucrose pellets. You can dissolve the sucrose Arnica 30c pellets in a small glass of water and place drops of the water in the mouth.
- *Hypericum 30c*: For extreme nerve pain after dental work, take doses of Hypericum 30c. This homeopathic remedy is classic for nerve pain

and/or injury. For severe pain, take a dose every one-to-two hours. Reduce the frequency as pain diminishes.

- *Nux vomica 30c* can also help reduce nerve pain and sensitivity after dental work. If you do not respond to Hypericum 30c within a day, try Nux vomica 30c every one-to-three hours. Repeat the remedy as needed, i.e., when pain worsens after having improved for a period of time.

CHAPTER 5

For Kids Only

Kids have incredible vitality. The Chinese describe children as having lots of *qi* and *yang* energy—the warming, heating, activating qualities in the body. This high level of energy means that kids tend to develop symptoms more quickly and dramatically, and they also tend to recover more swiftly and easily.

This section will guide you in choosing medicines from the Green Medicine chest that will enhance your child's natural vitality, to help them rebalance more quickly when confronted with acute illnesses.

You will find treatment suggestions for chronic conditions that require special attention, e.g., bed-wetting. You will also discover information about choices that will affect your child's long-term health and development, such as food introduction, vaccinations and media exposure.

Dosing herbs for acute illnesses

Liquid herbal preparations, such as teas and tinctures, usually are the easiest form of herbs for kids to take. Most tinctures are made with grain alcohol, which can be too strong for a child's sensitive mouth—young children have many more taste buds than adults! Many companies now offer kid-friendly tinctures made with glycerin rather than alcohol. Glycerin preparations extract slightly different constituents from plants than alcohol does. All in all, the two preparations are very similar, and the glycerin tinctures are much better tasting than tinctures prepared with alcohol.

- Ages 12 and older: full adult dose
  - Tea: 8 ounces of tea, made with 1 heaping teaspoon of herb(s) per cup of boiling water. Drink one cup, four-to-six times per day.

- Tincture: two (2) dropperfuls OR 40 drops of tincture every 2-to-4 hours
- Dried herb: two capsules every 2-to-4 hours

- Age 6: half the adult dosage
  - Tea: 4 ounces of tea, four-to-six times per day.
  - Tincture: one (1) dropperful OR 20 drops every 2-to-4 hours
  - Dried herb: one (1) capsule every 2-to-4 hours

- Age 3: one-quarter the adult dosage
  - Tea: 2 ounces of tea, four-to-six times per day
  - Tincture: 10 drops every 2-to-4 hours
  - Dried herb: 1 capsule, opened and stirred into water, juice, or food every 4 hours

- Age 1: one-sixth the adult dosage
  - Tea: 1 ounce every 2-to-4 hours
  - Tincture: 7-to-8 drops every 2-to-4 hours
  - Dried herb: one capsule opened and stirred into juice, water, or food. Give small sips or tastes of food every hour.

- For breastfeeding mothers: Drink tea or take a tincture for the quickest pass-through into the milk. Take full, adult doses and ingest herbs 30-to-45 minutes before nursing to ensure peak levels in the milk.

Essential oils for children

Because essential oils are so concentrated, you need to be mindful about which essential oils you use with children. See the list below for guidance about which oils are safe for different age groups.

Remember that essential oils are best "diluted" in a vegetable oil, rather than applied directly to the skin. The palms of the hands and the soles of the feet are the most absorptive skin surfaces. I often apply diluted essential oils to the bottom of my boys' feet, especially at bedtime, to maximize absorption.

Children, in general, have extremely sensitive skin, so use the essential oils sparingly, whether you are applying as skin oil or adding to bathwater mixed with milk (to disperse the oil in the water).

- Babies (birth to 18 months): rose, lavender, roman chamomile. Use 1/6 the adult dosage.

- Ages 18 months-to-4 four years old: the above list plus mandarin, tangerine, tea tree, *Eucalyptus radiata* (NOT the more common *Eucalyptus globulus,* which is a stronger, more stimulating oil). Use ¼ adult dosage
- Ages 5-to-12 years old: the above lists plus spearmint and other citruses (e.g., grapefruit, orange). Use ½ adult dosage

BED-WETTING

Some children's kidneys and bladder simply do not develop the "signal" in the nervous system to wake themselves at night when they need to urinate. This aspect of the nervous system may not fully mature until the late teens or early twenties.

Bed-wetting, or enuresis, can be embarrassing for children and frustrating for parents. I have a couple of patients in their teens who are unable to have sleepovers with friends because of bed-wetting.

You can take preventative measures that will minimize bed-wetting. In addition, I would encourage you to seek help from certain Classical Medicine providers who have treatment options to support your child.

- Approach bed-wetting as matter-of-factly as possible. Chastising your child, or calling him a "baby," won't help the situation. Most kids are deeply embarrassed and would prefer *not* to wet the bed. Rarely do kids choose to sleep in a pool of urine as a way of "acting out."
- Allow your child to continue wearing pull-ups as long as necessary. After changing one of my boys' beds almost nightly for a month during one of our "dry bed" campaigns, I was ready to return to pull-ups. Using the pull-ups does reduce the "signal" of lying in a wet bed. Having to change and wash sheets on an almost daily basis, however, may be a strain for parents. Remember to keep your stress levels in the equation too.
- Praise and encourage your child when she has a dry night. Make few or no comments on wet nights.
- If your child has a history of bed-wetting, consider taking pull-ups when you travel. Often children will "regress" developmentally when they are stressed, and travel certainly can strain a child. Other stressful situations can also trigger the return of bed-wetting, e.g., moving, the birth of a new sibling and/or the death of a family member.
- Reduce fluids after 5 p.m. You certainly don't want to dehydrate your child. A small amount of water (1/2 cup maximum) can wet a dry mouth.

- Wake your child to urinate before you go to sleep. For severe cases, you may also want to set the alarm for the middle of the night and take your child to the bathroom a second time.

- You can find devices to place in the bed that will buzz or ring when the child begins to wet the bed. The aim is to teach the body to pay attention to the "full bladder" signal. These work very well for some children; they traumatize others.

- From Chinese medical perspective, the inability to hold urine is a sign of "weakness in the lower gate," i.e., the "gate" that controls urine. Kidney *qi* and *jing* deficiency may also influence nocturnal enuresis. This does *not* mean that the kidney is diseased; instead, it suggests that the vitality of the kidney is diminished, making it more difficult for the kidney to fulfill its usual functions, including regulating the flow of urine. Work with a trained Chinese medical herbalist who can prescribe a botanical formula appropriate for your child, to rebuild kidney *qi* and *jing*. Blue Poppy Herbs offers "Dry Nites," the classical Chinese formula Bu Zhong Yi Qi Tan Jia Wei prepared as a glycerite tincture.

- Acupuncture can also strengthen kidney and bladder function. A Chinese practitioner likely would also be building the kidney and "spleen" (more accurately translated spleen, small intestine and pancreas) and digestive function, because the spleen governs the absorption of food, the foundation of energy and strength in the body, as well as muscle tone in the body.

- Constitutional homeopathic treatment can also address the root of bed-wetting. Work with a trained "classical" homeopath who can prescribe a constitutional homeopathic remedy, or possibly a series of remedies, to address the underlying root of your child's bed-wetting. In homeopathy there is no one remedy for bed-wetting. Several remedies can help; the classical homeopath will choose the one best-suited for your child.

- Flower essences can be very helpful to address the shame and/or distress your child may have about bed-wetting. Consider some of the following:

  - Buttercup – feeling worthless or unimportant
  - Larch – fear of making a mistake; paralyzed by fear of being ridiculed or shamed by others; self-censoring
  - Pine – self-criticism, self-blame; feeling one's life is a failure

- Pink Monkeyflower: fear someone will discover something terrible; profound shame

COLIC

Your baby's digestive tract is just developing. In this pristine state, mom's milk really is the best and only food for your infant. Even mom's milk, though, may contain constituents that irritate the baby's digestive tract. You can work with several approaches to settle his or her digestive tract. Infants, generally, respond quickly to changes; you should know in a short period of time if a particular approach is working.

Be sure to rule out any possible organic causes of colic, such as bowel obstruction or lactose intolerance. Any major problems usually become apparent from a couple of days to a week after birth.

- Nurse when both you and the baby are relaxed. Trying to nurse amidst remodeling carpenters or on a bus at rush hour is *not* conducive to milk drop for mom or easy digestion for the baby. Drink chamomile or hops tea (hops also increases breast milk production), play relaxing music and make your environment as relaxed as possible when you nurse. When either you or the baby are stressed or irritated, blood is shunted away from the digestive tract, in favor of the muscles, lungs and heart. The digestive tract obviously cannot function well in these conditions.
- Massage the baby's stomach a couple of times a day. When suffering with colic, the baby probably will not respond well to a firm massage, particularly right after eating. Wait a few minutes; then, begin a soft, rhythmic massage of the abdomen, moving in gentle clockwise circles (up the baby's right side and down his left). This gentle massage encourages the baby's normal digestive movement.
- Essential oils can also help relax the digestive system. Remember that only three essential oils are safe for use with babies: lavender, roman chamomile and rose. Of these three, lavender is the most appropriate to soothe the digestive tract. Babies have extremely sensitive skin. Watch for any signs of reaction to the oil and immediately discontinue use if you notice any kind of skin reaction. In general, do not use a particular essential oil for more than a week. Ongoing, continual use of a particular essential oil increases the possibility of developing a reaction or sensitivity to the oil. After a week of use, take a week off OR

substitute a different oil (e.g., roman chamomile). At this age, babies do not have many oils to choose from. The best strategy is to take a week off and then resume using the essential oil, if necessary.

- Remove anything from your diet that may irritate the baby's digestive tract. Some of the most common gas-producing and/or irritating foods include: brassica-family vegetables (cabbage, cauliflower, broccoli, kale, kohlrabi, Brussels sprouts); garlic; onions; and for some children, any non-human milk, e.g., goat, cow, or sheep. If removing these foods still does not correct the baby's colic, consider specialized testing (see information about food intolerances and allergies) to detect which specific foods are irritating the baby's digestive tract. Remove these from your diet, as these foods do "pass through" your milk.

- Drinking chamomile or other soothing, nervine teas half an hour before nursing is perfect timing for these herbs to assimilate into the breast milk. Nervine teas calm as well as feed the nervous system. By "feed" I do NOT mean stimulate. Many nervine teas, for example, contain calcium and other nutrients that support the nervous system. These teas will calm but not sedate the nervous system.

- Breast-feed children as long as possible. Developing infant digestive and immune systems are not able to handle solid foods until at least six months of age. Many children develop food intolerances because of early exposure to food other than human breast milk. Recent research links adult-onset diabetes with early exposure to cow's milk (see information below on food introduction).

- Smaller, more frequent feedings.

- Skin-to-skin contact can soothe and calm the infant, helping the digestive system to function more smoothly.

- Breast-feeding mothers may experiment with eliminating certain foods to discover any foods that are irritating the infant. Cabbage, caffeine, onions, garlic and highly spiced foods are common irritants. Laxatives, such as large amounts of prune juice (more than one cup per day), also may irritate the baby's digestive system.

- Feed your baby in a quiet, relaxed environment whenever possible.

- Slippery elm is a good food substitute for extreme cases of colic, acting as a demulcent to soothe the infant's digestive tract. Mix two tablespoons of slippery-elm-bark powder with a small amount of sweetener (maple syrup or molasses). Add hot water or hot milk—mother's milk, if you are still breast- feeding—until the mixture is the consistency of porridge. Feed the baby slippery elm in place of other solid foods.

Botanical medicines

- For breast-feeding mothers, drink chamomile tea to soothe the infant's digestive system.
- For children receiving formula, add 1/4 cup chamomile tea to a bottle of formula.
- Aromatic seeds have a soothing effect on the digestive system. Prepare an infusion of one of the following seeds (one teaspoon of seed per cup of water): cardamom, fennel, anise or cumin. Strain and add 1/4 cup to infant's formula, or drink a cup of this tea 20-to-30 minutes before breast-feeding.

Physical therapy:

Gently massage the infant's abdomen with a good vegetable oil (e.g., sesame, almond or other cold-pressed oil) in a clockwise, circular motion.

Homeopathic remedies 30c potency

- Magnesium phosphorica – cramping pain that improves with warm applications
- Chamomilla – child is extremely irritable, wants to be carried, then demands to be put down. Inconsolable. One cheek is red, the other pale.
- Colocynthis – cramping, abdominal pain that is relieved by pressure and by drawing the knees toward the chest
- Bryonia – feels worse following the slightest motion; generally irritable

When to consult a physician:

- If the infant is losing weight
- If colic routinely disturbs the infant's sleep cycle

DIAPER RASH

Most diaper rashes are caused by prolonged exposure to wet, soiled diapers. A dry bottom decreases the chances of developing diaper rash.

General recommendations:

- Change diapers frequently, right after each bowel movement.
- Expose baby's bottom to light and air as often as possible.

- Use cotton diapers without plastic pants whenever possible; cotton breathes more than plastic-coated diapers. Use wool "soakers" instead of plastic pants.
- Apply calendula ointment and/or dust with calendula powder. Calendula promotes skin healing and has antibacterial action.
- Use arrowroot powder or bentonite clay instead of commercial baby powders.
- Use olive oil instead of Vaseline® or commercial ointments, which have chemical additives that may irritate the baby's skin.
- Wash diapers with soap flakes. Avoid harsh detergents. Add vinegar to the final rinse water and dry diapers in the sunshine if possible.

For severe rashes:

- Apply comfrey-root ointment to the diaper rash. Comfrey leaf does not contain as much allantoin, the active constituent that promotes skin healing.
- Apply Calendula ointment, which also promotes skin healing.
- Avoid ointments with goldenseal, as this herb may irritate sensitive tissue in the genital area.

When to consult a physician

- If you have tried the above suggestions and the rash has persisted for more than a week
- If the skin is raw or bleeding

EARACHE

Earaches are especially common in children, in large part because the developing Eustachian tubes do not effectively drain the ear. Whether young or old, the pain associated with ear infections is usually intense and requires immediate care.

The best treatment is prevention. Many children respond well to dietary changes. Eliminating dairy and sugar reduces mucus-forming foods; dairy and wheat are the two most common food allergens in North America. Sometimes removing these three foods—milk, sugar and wheat—is enough to stop recurrent ear infections.

Most children with chronic ear infections are caught on a merry-go-round of antibiotic treatments. The antibiotics clear the infection, but another quickly follows, usually within four-to-six weeks. Antibiotics wipe out the good bacteria in the body, as well as the invading bacteria in the ear. After antibiotic treatment, the body is more susceptible to infection.

Keeping the ears warm and covered when outdoors also helps prevent ear infections, as does increasing vitamin C during the cold season. For children, 500 mg of vitamin C twice per day is an adequate dosage. Adults may supplement one (1) gram three-to-five times per day.

The following suggestions are for acute ear infections, when preventive measures have not succeeded:

General recommendations

Sit the patient near a 120-watt light bulb, with the ear close enough to feel warmth, but not close enough to cause burning. Carefully monitor. The warmth will soothe ear pain and increase circulation in the area, which brings more immune cells to fight the infection.

Hydrotherapy:

- Alternate hot and cold applications to the ear. Wring out a washcloth in water as hot as you can stand and apply for five minutes to the ear. Follow with a cold application (a wet washcloth put in the freezer, or a bag of frozen peas) for one minute. Repeat the cycle, alternating hot and cold, at least three times. Always end with a cold application.
- Wet-socks treatment at bedtime (see "Hydrotherapy" section, Chapter 2).
- Constitutional hydrotherapy treatment once per day (see "Hydrotherapy" section, Chapter 2).

Botanical therapy:

- Oil of mullein and/or garlic – Place two or three drops of gently warmed oil in the ear. (Warm the oil by placing the bottle in a bowl of hot water for a couple of minutes.) Mullein oil reduces pain and inflammation. Both garlic and mullein have antimicrobial action. CAUTION: Use ear drops only if the tympanic membrane (eardrum) is not broken.
- Echinacea and goldenseal tincture or capsules—Dose according to age (see above)

Homeopathic remedies: 30c potency

- Aconite – Earache begins after exposure to cold, dry wind. Bright red ears, high fever, sudden onset. Very sensitive to noise. Sharp pain. Anxious, restless. Thirst for cold drinks. Onset after shock.
- Belladonna – sudden, violent onset. Dilated pupils. Throbbing blood vessels in the neck. Pain causes delirium. Child may have nightmares and call out in sleep. Throbbing, shooting, sharp pains. No thirst with fever. Red-hot throbbing ear.
- Chamomilla – irritable; intense pain. One cheek is red, the other pale. The child wants to be held and carried, yet arches her back. Inconsolable. Earaches from teething. Grass-green stool.
- Ferrum phos – first stage of infection, before pus develops. Pulsating, throbbing pain. Flushed face. High fever with few symptoms. Use when Belladonna fails.
- Hepar sulph – mucus, pus in ear. For later stage of infection, when pus has developed behind the eardrum. Hates drafts, wants to cover ears or head. Chilly, oversensitive, sweats easily. Feels better with hot, damp weather.
- Pulsatilla – for a "ripe" (second or third stage) cold and ear infection. Copious, thick, yellow-green discharge. Changing symptoms. No thirst. Feels better in fresh, cold, open air; worse in warm, stuffy room. Feels worse in the evening.

When to consult a physician:

- If ear infections occur more than once or twice in a year
- If ear infection and pain persist for more than four days
- If ear infection is accompanied by a high fever (above 102°F)
- If the child has a stiff neck or arches the back
- If the ear oozes pus or blood
- If redness or swelling develops in the bony area behind the ear

FOOD INTRODUCTION

Two of the most common questions parents ask me are, "When should I start giving my baby solid food?" and "What should I feed her?" The answers to these questions have varied from decade to decade. Fifty years ago pediatricians recommended eating rice cereal at six weeks. Some physicians now recommend nothing but breast milk for the first year. Thankfully, your baby will tell you when he is ready for food.

Some parents take pride in feeding their babies a wide variety of foods at an early age. I cringe when parents tell me their three-month old is already eating "table food." Why is it important to wait before introducing solid foods?

Infants' digestive tracts are immature and develop slowly. At about 6 months of age, the infant begins to produce digestive enzymes needed for the breakdown of different foods. Immune globulin A (IgA), which is a protective immune globulin, just begins to line the digestive tract at about seven months of age. Before this age, the infant's digestive tract has no protection at all against allergenic substances, which is why I recommend introducing hypoallergenic foods first.

Most importantly, pay attention to your child's cues. Unless your baby has a special medical condition, you do not need to rush introducing solid food. Your baby will know just the right time to begin eating, just as he or she will know when to crawl, walk and talk.

Watch for the following cues to signal that he or she is ready to try food:

- Is she sitting up by herself? Babies can swallow milk while lying down, but they need to be upright to swallow solid foods.
- Does he show interest in food? Is he trying to grab food on the table, or from your hand?
- Is she teething? Teeth signal that the body is ready for solid food.
- When you feed your baby, does he swallow, or does he thrust the food back out with his tongue? The tongue thrusting reflex begins to diminish at six-to-seven months of age. This physical mechanism prevents infants from choking. If your child is spitting the food out, hold off for a while and then try again.

Once you know your child is ready, the next question is, "What do I feed him?"

Most physicians suggest avoiding common allergens such as wheat, cow's milk, oranges, eggs, sugar and chocolate for at least one year. Introduce one new food at a time, preferably no more frequently than every four days. Remember that food reactions can occur up to four days after ingesting a food. Watch for any signs of reaction:

- Runny nose
- Sneezing

- Wheezing
- Rashes and/or itchy skin
- Stool changes
- Red ring around the anus
- Diaper rash
- Sore mouth
- Personality and/or mood changes
- Changes in handwriting (older children), e.g., writing backwards or inverting numbers.

Once you know your child does not react to a food, offer it every five-to-six days. Eating the same foods day after day increases the likelihood of developing food reactions. Rotating foods minimizes the possibility of developing food sensitivities.

Above all, have fun! Mealtime should be pleasant for both of you. If it is not, consult with your doctor. Your child may not be ready or perhaps there are other issues that may need to be addressed to make eating an enjoyable experience.

Solid Food Introduction Schedule

6 months (approximately): 1-to-2 tablespoons/day

These are hypoallergenic, pureed, mashed foods containing iron. Focus on tasting foods.

Much of your baby's nutrition is still from breast milk. If any foods are too sweet, try again at about seven months.

brown rice cereal	blackberry
stewed prunes	pear
ground oatmeal	broccoli
cherry	peach
spinach	leafy greens
apricot	kiwi
Jerusalem artichoke	squash (summer and winter)
grape	yam
cauliflower	carrot

9 months: 2-to-4 tablespoons/day

These foods are high in zinc and good for the immune system. Be careful; some of these may be hard to digest. If so, wait a month and try again.

sweet potato	cabbage
lentils	apples
papaya	blueberry
avocado	potato
string bean	nectarine
split pea soup	millet

12 months: 4-to-10 tablespoons/day

peas	yogurt*
soy milk	parsnip
asparagus	wheat*
rice milk	barley
tofu*	eggs*
goat milk	juices**

*If soy, dairy, wheat or eggs are known allergens in the family, you may want to avoid these at this point and monitor carefully for allergic reactions.

**Dilute juices with at least 50% water. Give juices only as a treat and not as regular part of the diet. Extractor juices (like those sold in grocery stores or made with extractor juicers, such as the Champion juicer) are simply too sugary. One glass of apple juice, for example, is made from five apples. A child can easily drink a glass of juice, but would she be able to eat five apples? If you use a Vitamix or other whole food juicer that does not create a pulp, you can give the juice undiluted.

18 months

beets	lamb*
kelp	tahini
beet greens	turkey*
rye	beans
(legumes)	chicken*
rutabaga	

*If your child will be vegetarian, check with your doctor to make sure he or she is eating the right foods for sufficient protein and B-vitamins.

21 months

almond butter	eggplant
pineapple	orange
banana	cashew butter
grapefruit	brewer's yeast
walnut	

2-3 years

sunflower seed	cottage cheese
peanut butter	cow's milk

Cow's milk and your child's health

Genetic researchers consider northern Europeans' ability to digest milk throughout their life cycle a genetic aberration or adaptation rather than the norm. On a global scale, most of us can digest milk only until age two or three, and human milk is the milk of choice. Each animal's milk stimulates different types of growth. Human milk, for instance, is high in essential fatty acids and stimulates brain and neural development. In contrast, a baby calf's first priority is to stand and walk, so cow's milk stimulates muscle development.

A note on cow's milk: The following extensive research, which demonstrates that early introduction of cow's milk can increase the risk of developing diabetes later in life, is listed in the Appendices for further reference. (1,2) In genetically susceptible infants, exposure to cow's milk triggers the development of antibodies that destroy pancreatic beta cells, which are responsible for insulin production. Avoiding exposure to cow's milk during the first year may reduce the likelihood of developing diabetes later in life in these genetically susceptible infants. (3) A more recent study shows that consuming cow's milk throughout childhood doubles the risk for developing diabetes. The study included children up to 14 years of age. (4)

The American Dairy Council has been very effective in convincing us that young children need milk. If you look globally, most humans cannot digest dairy products, from any animal, after age two or three. Northern European people, especially Scandinavians, have developed the ability to digest milk products after that age. This genetic adaptation occurred over hundreds of years, likely because of the limited number of foods available that far north, especially during the winter. The farther you go from northern Europe, the more difficulty people have digesting dairy products.

Estimated Percentage of Lactose Intolerance in Different Populations(7)

Vietnamese	100%
American Indian	95%
Southern Italian	72%
African American	65%
Northern Italian	50%
French	32%
White Americans	22%
Austrian	20%
Northern European	7%
Dutch	0%

Unless you have a child with pure Scandinavian genetic heritage, I would encourage you not to introduce cow's milk at all.

As a teenager I worked at a YMCA camp that hired international counselors. One day, while I was in the kitchen, Ahmed, a counselor from Lebanon, watched me refilling milk containers.

"I do not understand you Americans," he said, shaking his head. "You eat baby food. *Baby* food. No one in my country drinks milk after they are weaned."

I think of him often when I see the American Dairy Council posters, "Got milk?" No, I don't have milk and neither do my children. We get plenty of calcium and other nutrients from our diet, even without the addition of cow's milk.

INFANT MASSAGE

Touch is an important "nutrient" for infants. Gentle, regular touch stimulates both physical and neural development. Touch-deprived infants suffer from a range of developmental abnormalities.

One of my patients, now a sturdy 13-year-old, was born without eyeballs. Kevin also had surgery to correct a defect in his stomach a few days after birth. In Hong Kong, a baby with a birth defect is considered a shameful blight on the family. Kevin's parents left him in the hospital and never returned.

As an infant, Kevin was left to lie on his left side for most of his first year. The only touch Kevin received was from nurses who came to bottle feed him or change his soiled diapers. At the end of his first year, Kevin began a merry-go-round of orphanages that continued until he was three years old. Thankfully, a caregiver in one of the orphanages bonded with the boy and adopted him a couple of years later.

Today Kevin has very poorly developed speech. After years of intensive work, he can articulate about 10 words clearly. If he had had normal touch stimulation, he likely would have completely normal speech today. The lack of touch, combined with changes in his skull shape from being left to lie in one position through all of his first year, permanently altered some of his brain function. His adoptive parents have taken extraordinary measures and reversed some of the early deprivation. Sadly, though, the early lack of touch left devastating, permanent changes in his neural development.

Instructions for baby massage

Choose a quiet, warm room. If you have a bath scheduled, bathe your baby first.

Place a baby blanket or soft towel on the floor. Pour a small amount of vegetable oil in your hand. Weleda calendula oil is my first choice. Plain olive oil is also a wonderful choice. You can add one drop of rose or lavender essential oil, two of the only essential oils safe for use with infants. Add a drop of essential oil to one tablespoon of pure vegetable oil. Rub your hands together to warm the oil.

Begin with the hands. Gently make circles in the palm of the baby's hand and then slowly, carefully work up the arm. Make small circles at the back of the neck. Smooth your fingers over the forehead and make gentle circles over the cheeks. This face massage is particularly helpful during teething, when the gums are sore. The jaws may also be sore from the effort of nursing and/or eating.

Make small, gentle circles over the chest and then move down to the abdomen. The large intestine naturally moves up the baby's right side, across the top of the abdomen and down the baby's left side. Of course, you will be looking at a mirror image of the baby. Imagine that the belly is the face of a clock that you are looking at. Move *clockwise* around the baby's abdomen. This can be very soothing for colicky babies.

Move now to the feet. Make circles on the bottom of the feet. Gently move up the legs, toward the abdomen. Always massage *toward* the heart, to encourage circulation. For an infant, even the softest of movements will still encourage blood circulation.

Finish with gentle rocking and snuggling.

Infant massage helps the baby to relax and come to know its physical body in a relaxed, pleasurable environment. So much of a baby's experience is defined by discomfort, i.e., wet diapers, hunger and cold. Massage offers your baby an opportunity to come to know his or her body through joy and relaxation, rather than discomfort.

These massages are for you, too. After hours of struggling to meet the baby's needs, these peaceful minutes are pure gold for your soul too. Remember that the more peaceful you are, the more relaxed your baby can be. Your physical, mental and emotional state are the "umbilical cord" that continues to feed (or disrupt) your newborn.

INSOMNIA

Bless you if you are a parent struggling with a child or children with disrupted sleep. My twin boys did not sleep through the night until they were 30 months old. By then, I was severely sleep-deprived. Sleep problems may cause mild upsets for some children, but they are VERY disruptive for parents.

When your child is young, even during infancy, develop a regular sleep routine. Regularity soothes most children, even if they resist the routine. I use the words "routine" or "rhythm" because you may not be able to keep the exact same clock time each evening. Aim to be as consistent with time as possible; the regular rhythm will also support the children in preparing for bed.

Consider incorporating some or all of the following suggestions for soothing your child into sleep. Keep in mind that your approach likely will need to change over time. Just when you are certain you have the perfect system, your child may hit another bump in the road and enter another period of restless sleep. This is a fairly normal pattern, since the nervous, endocrine and immune systems go through maturation spurts. Take a deep breath, put on your thinking cap, and plug in your intuition. Approaches that worked in the past may not be effective now, or methods that had no effect when she was younger may work like a charm now. Be open to experimenting to discover a "new norm."

- Warm baths can be very soothing to prepare for bedtime.
- Add 1-to-3 drops of essential oils, mixed with 1 tablespoon of milk (the fat and protein in the milk helps disperse the essential oil in the bath water). For babies, roman chamomile and lavender are safe choices. See the beginning of the chapter for a list of child-safe essential oils.
- Massage your child after the bath. In a warm room, lay a towel or blanket on the floor. Use pure vegetable oils, e.g., olive or almond, that is room temperature or slightly warm. Weleda makes wonderful calendula oil for babies. Massage in small, gentle circles, always mov-

ing toward the heart. Rub the abdomen in a smooth, clockwise circle—the direction the intestines naturally move.

- A teaspoon of barley malt syrup at bedtime deeply soothes some children.

- Nurse infants to sleep: I nursed the boys to sleep until they were almost two years old. Some specialists recommend disassociating nursing and sleep, for your own sanity. You will have to assess your particular situation and your child's needs. Some children simply refuse to nurse at a certain age. The mother may feel deeply rejected. The child often is asserting his or her independence. VERY occasionally, the mother's breast may be diseased, e.g., with breast cancer. This is a rare occurrence. If your baby rejects the nipple at a young age, please have your breasts evaluated, just to be on the safe side. Most likely you simply have an independent child.

- For breast-feeding mothers, drink hops or chamomile tea a couple of hours before bedtime. The soothing, relaxing properties of the tea will pass through the breast milk to your child.

- Avoid putting the child to bed with a bottle, particularly one filled with juice. Leaving juice or milk in contact with the baby's mouth all night can contribute to cavity formation.

- Say prayers and/or sing a song as you tuck your child into bed. Regular repetition of a soothing song or words helps your child to shift into relaxation. When the boys were very young, I used to lie down between them and hold their hands as they fell asleep.

- Play quiet, relaxing music, e.g., Native American flute music, "New Age" relaxation music, or gentle classical music.

- For older children, from toddler through elementary school, consider listening to the bedtime stories of Jim Weiss, "Good Night." These lovely recorded stories (fun for adults, too!) guide children into a relaxed state and prepare them to sleep.

- Keep the house quiet; dim the lights. If possible, move adult conversations and other sound into a different part of the house.

- The calmer you are, the calmer your children will be. Make sure that you are as relaxed and rested as possible. Arrange to sleep at a friend or another family member's home once a week so that you have at least one night of uninterrupted sleep. This will increase your own patience and tolerance with your child, when you enter the day more rested.

TEETHING

Many symptoms may accompany the eruption of teeth in an infant, including colds, ear infections and diarrhea. The following suggestions are meant specifically for the gum and mouth symptoms.

- Soak a clean cloth in chamomile tea, wring out and place in the freezer. Give to baby to chew on when he or she shows signs of discomfort.
- Water-filled plastic "teething rings" can soothe inflamed gums, but they also contain Bisphenol A (BPA), a plasticizer that has xenoestrogen effects. "*Xeno*" means "foreign," so xenoestrogens are chemicals foreign to the body that stimulate estrogen receptor sites in the body. The clear plastics used to make teething rings and baby bottles contain BPA. Tiny amounts migrate from the plastic into the baby, but research by the Consumers Union shows that even one part per *billion* affected animals in the study. Edward (Ned) Groth III, Ph.D., a senior scientist at Consumers Union, explains that ". . . the effect that is of concern here is a disruption of the developmental process. This could affect intelligence. It could affect behavior. It could affect learning ability. It could affect reproductive ability, fertility many years after the exposure occurs."
- If you are breast-feeding, drink chamomile and oat straw tea (equal parts). The herbs will pass into the breast milk.

Homeopathic remedies 30c potency

- Calcarea carbonica – late dentition (teeth slow to emerge). Fontanelles slow to close. Ear infections sometimes accompany teething.
- Chamomilla – a classic remedy for teething, especially for inconsolable children, or children who are extremely irritable and demand to be carried, yet arch their back away from whomever is carrying them. One cheek is red, the other pale. Grassy green, runny stools may accompany teething.
- Ignatia – child is distressed, but not as irritable as in previous case. The baby sobs, sighs and cries. The whole body— or single body parts— may tremble.

TELEVISION

I grew up with television, the electronic babysitter of my generation. My parents never limited or monitored our television viewing. I have memories of watching the turmoil after Martin Luther King's and Bobby Kennedy's assassinations and the war in Vietnam. The sixties entered my fledgling life and mind through the flickering black-and-white images on the TV.

By the time I was 11 years old, I was too busy with music and other activities to watch TV. By default I watched the evening news, because the TV was on continuously in the kitchen. Otherwise, I did not watch the sit-coms and other programs many high school students waited for in the evening. At first I didn't have time; then, I lost interest.

For my own children, I've chosen to limit television watching. That decision was based, in part, on my own experience, bolstered by research on the effects of watching television for prolonged periods of time.

In 2009, children ages 2-to-5 spent an average of *32 hours a week* watching television, DVDs, DVR and videos and using game consoles. Kids ages 6-to-11 spent about 28 hours a week in front of the TV. The children spent the vast majority of that time (97 percent) viewing live television.

The American Academy of Pediatrics suggests the following limits for television watching:

- Birth to 2 years old: ZERO hours of television per day
- Ages 2-to-6: one hour of television per day
- Ages 6-to-12: a maximum of two hours per day

Before their permanent teeth erupt, young children live in an imaginative, dream-like world. The edges of reality are malleable, blurred. Television weighs equally with family gatherings and other social activities in their lives.

Linda, a colleague with two young children, reported that her four-year-old son had been watching an old Western movie with John Wayne.

"Indians are bad, Mommy," said her son when she walked into the room.

"What do you mean, John?"

"They're bad, Mommy, aren't they?"

"What makes you think that?"

"Because the cowboys are the good guys."

"Wait a minute," said Linda, "let's talk about this. Do you understand that TV is not real?"

Her son looked puzzled. "Of course it's real, Mommy."

Linda shook her head. "No, John, TV is NOT real. Most of TV is made up. That's important for you to understand."

John's response is typical for preschoolers who are unable to discern imagination from reality. During this formative stage, children are developing their sense of themselves and the world around them. They form many opinions and prejudices about the world, based on their experiences. In their minds, television "experience" weighs just as heavily as day-to-day interactions.

"When a young child sees somebody being shot, stabbed, raped, brutalized, degraded, or murdered on TV," explain Lt. Colonel Dave Grossman and Gloria DeGaetano, authors of *Stop Teaching our Kids to Kill* (Crown Publishers, 1999), "to them it is as though it is actually happening. Imagine children of three, four, or five watching 'splatter' movies in which they spend sixty minutes learning to relate to a cast of characters and then in the last sixty minutes of the movie they watch helplessly as their newfound friends are hunted down and brutally murdered. This is the moral and psychological equivalent of introducing a child to a group of new friends, letting them play with those friends and then butchering them in front of the child." (p. 55)

The effects of electronic technology

But what about all of those wonderful educational programs—Sesame Street, Bob the Builder, Barney and a host of other children's programs? Yes, many of these programs offer valuable information and insights. They teach skills like social interactions and sometimes movement and songs, IF the child will actually get up and move with the adults and kids on the screen, which is a rarity. The television does NOT teach children to move or interact. The television by nature encourages a child to watch passively, without interacting.

Rudolph Steiner, who developed the Waldorf educational system, believed that young children learn best by imitation, and he encouraged the preschool and kindergarten teachers to model activities children could emulate. In addition, he believed in stimulating children's imaginations. Instead of giving them plastic toys that replicated household objects, he filled the preschool and kindergarten rooms with natural objects the children could use to project their imaginations.

Pine cones, for example, became eggs cooking on the stove. Acorns were beans and rice, served on a "plate" of cut sections of a log. Stones, shells, silk scarves and simple wooden blocks filled the play area. When I worked in a Waldorf Kindergarten, I loved watching the children transform these simple, natural objects into stores, castles, railroad stations, buses and kitchens.

Offering the children too many slick, shiny toys robs them of the opportunity to transform simple objects into endless universes of imagination. I notice my boys rarely use toys for their intended purposes. The hydraulic construction set, for example, soon becomes pieces for "fences" on a horse ranch; the chemistry set becomes the ingredients for a wizard's spells; the magic set has transfigured into endless games of star exploration and alien encounters. The list goes on and on. Instead of encouraging them to use the set only for its intended purpose, I'm delighted that they metamorphose the pieces for other uses.

Television moves children even further from the roots of their imagination than plastic replicas of daily objects. The television does not have *anything* tactile for the child to manipulate. This physical contact helps to mold the child's experience of the world and literally shapes the brain. Passively watching the television, expecting it to do everything for us, bypasses these important developmental steps of learning to touch and interact with the world.

Slow play

Watching many hours of television robs children of time otherwise spent playing outside, reading and creating their own imaginary games. This "slow play," according to Katherine Luiten, childhood occupational therapist and parenting coach, develops the frontal lobe of the brain, where higher thinking processes such as problem solving and reflective thinking occur. In contrast, sitting in front of the television or a video game bombards the brain with images that change every 3-to-5 seconds. This hyper-stimulation of the lower brain stem triggers the "fight or flight" response. When the lower brain stem is hyper-stimulated, attention span decreases.

Remember that children up to 6 or 7 years of age learn primarily through imitation. And what does TV offer for them to imitate?

If they are watching television, even cartoons supposedly geared for children, they are being exposed to extremely high levels of violence:

- A preschooler who watches about two hours of cartoons a day is exposed to nearly 10,000 violent episodes each year. At least 500 of them feature a potent set of contextual features, making them a high risk for teaching aggressive attitudes and behaviors.
- Nearly 40 percent of all the violent incidents on television are initiated by characters that possess qualities that make them attractive role models to kids. More than half of these incidents feature physical aggression that would be lethal or incapacitating if it were to occur in real life.
- By age 18, a typical American child will have seen at least 200,000 dramatized acts of violence and 40,000 screen murders.

(page 49, Stop Teaching Our Kids to Kill.)

Video games teach children the skills of firing, often with plastic guns, so that they can actually control and perform the murders on the screen. Many of these video games feature the same technology used by the U.S. Army to teach sharp-shooting skills. Psychologists point out that a soldier (or a murderer, the civilian equivalent) needs three components: a gun, the skill to use the gun and the will to kill. These battle simulation games provide the skill and the will to kill.

These video games also have addictive qualities. Children report that 60 percent of the time they play the video games longer than they intended.

Why are these games so seductive? The games automatically adjust to the child's skill level, meaning the child experiences instant success and immediate gratification. She never has to struggle with the challenges of the "real" world, grappling with developing skills that may be out of her reach. She also operates in a virtual world that appears to be completely in her control. Together, these factors seduce children to enter an illusory world of control and satisfaction.

Your Brain on Television

"Slow" play, such as reading, playing ball, digging holes in the garden and coloring, develops the frontal lobe, which governs attention span, problem-solving skills, decision-making and impulse control. Children who spend hours a day watching television or playing video games do not engage in the "slow" play activities that stimulate the frontal lobe. Instead, television and video games hyper-stimulate the brain stem and the "fight or flight" response.

Katherine Luiten points out that the frontal lobe develops slowly, reaching peak maturation at about 24-to-25-years-old for women and 25-to-26-years-old for men.

"For kids who have spent years 'plugged in,'" explains Luiten, "they can't suddenly wake up and decide to abandon television and make up for that lost 'slow play' time. They need years to fully develop the frontal lobe. It can be done, but it takes a long time."

Luiten also points out that many children are multi-tasking while they study. They listen to music, watch TV, text friends and surf the net while they are reading and studying.

"The truth is that the brain *can't* multi-task," says Luiten. "We can only pay attention to one thing at a time. The brain focuses on one activity and ignores the rest. Kids who are multi-tasking while they study only retain information for a short time. From studies we know they don't remember anything from their study time a few months later."

Technology and family time

As our culture becomes increasingly dependent on television for entertainment, we have less and less time face-to-face, actually talking and communicating with one another. We sit side-by-side on the sofa, with our attention directed straight ahead at our "entertainment center." We become passive observers rather than active participants interacting with one another. Like worshippers at church, we pay homage to the beloved box (or now, flat TV screen), devoting our full attention to its homily.

Many of us have lost the ability to entertain ourselves. We expect the exterior world to amuse us. My ex-husband's parents bought an RV when they retired and traveled around the country sight-seeing. Dedicated TV watchers, they decided to visit one of the towns where "Gunsmoke" was filmed.

"There was nothing there," said Larry, clearly disgusted after their trip. "I mean *nothing*. Just a few buildings—no stores or museums. It was a wasted trip."

"Wasted," I thought, for someone who expects the world to entertain them. I probably would have delighted in the musty scent of sagebrush and the diamond blanket of desert night sky. That beauty, though, would be lost on Larry—unless, perhaps, he viewed it on a television screen.

Before the advent of television, radio revolutionized our communication. Although radio also smacks of passive entertainment, at least the mind is engaged in forming pictures. Radio engages the imagination, encouraging us to create or own mental landscapes. When traveling, I love to play books on tape or storytellers for the boys. I also enjoy creating mental pictures of the lands and characters described in the book. I often remember these stories much better than books made into movies, because I created the "movie" in my own mind.

Your family may discover a whole range of satisfying activities when you shut off the box. One family reported spending summer evenings watching the chickens in their back yard and delighting in the hens' antics. My boys and I play catch in the evening after dinner, or play a board game. Sometimes we do watch a movie, as a special treat. I also haul the television out of storage every couple of years to watch the Olympics. Otherwise, it gathers dust in the barn.

How can you woo children away from electronic media entertainment?

- Create and follow guidelines for television and other electronic media in your home.
- Limit time with all electronic devices (count total time for all devices, not just television):
  - Birth to age 2: NO time with electronic devices

- Ages 2-to-6: maximum one hour
- Ages 6-to-12: maximum 2 hours

- Carefully choose the programs you allow your child to watch. Make sure they finish their homework before they park themselves in front of the television. Consider choosing the programs you will watch at the beginning of the week. Stick to the schedule.

- If your children have behavioral problems, unplug your television and haul it to the thrift store. Discover other ways to spend time with your children. *365 Days Unplugged Family Fun Activities* (Adams Media Corp Publication, 1996) by Steve and Ruth Bennett offers a full year of daily activities to entertain and challenge children.

- Focus on reading and language skills. Reading develops the frontal lobe of the brain, a major component of dampening impulsive behavior.

- Read out loud to your children. I have read to my children since they were *in utero*. My boys and I have read several series of books since they were about three years old. I have enjoyed revisiting old favorites (e.g., Paddington Bear, the Narnia series, Winnie the Pooh and Henry Huggins). I've also discovered new "friends," e.g., Harry Potter; Ramona; and Jack and Annie, protagonists of the Magic Tree House series.

- Talk about the books you read together and the ones they are reading on their own. What do they think of these other children's adventures? Why do they think someone behaves in a certain way? How do the characters influence the world they live in? Would they make the same or different choices?

- Turn off the television during dinner. Revive the long lost art of conversation. Ask, "What was the best thing that happened today? What was the most difficult? What did you learn today?" Make sure *you* answer the questions, too.

- Turn off all electronic media during study time. Kids retain very little information when they are multi-tasking during study time.

- Sing and play music together. Even if you are not a musician, you can find wonderful collections of percussion instruments that allow you to make music in simple, fun ways. Music also develops the central cortex and stimulates other creative centers in the brain. See *The Ear and the Voice* (Rowman & Littlefield Publishers, 2004) by Alfred A. Tomatis and *Toddler Brain Basics 12 to 24 Months* by Brilliant Beginnings.

VACCINATIONS

Many parents ask me for advice about vaccinations. This is a difficult question for any parent, particularly because the social and medical systems in our country are designed to force parents to vaccinate children.

In truth, vaccinations were a huge breakthrough in medical technology. Before the development of the smallpox vaccine in 1796 by Dr. Edward Jenner in rural England, this disease had taken millions of lives on every continent. Polio also crippled or killed millions before Salk and Sabin developed the polio vaccine. Up until that time, we had a very hazy idea of how these diseases developed and how to prevent them. Vaccines truly have offered great gifts to humanity.

Enamored with the power of vaccines, however, we have overlooked the possible harm. Many of the current cases of polio are due to the use of live polio vaccine. In the 1950's, isolated, indigenous people were forced to take the smallpox vaccine. Despite this worldwide frenzy to vaccinate against smallpox, the Centers for Disease Control and Prevention (CDC) maintain samples of the smallpox virus. If we are so intent on eradicating the virus, why are we saving samples for posterity?

Human history is entwined with the diseases we face. The epidemic of one millennia or century, once "cured," gives way to another. Through the 1930's, the major feared "killer" in the U.S. was tuberculosis. My grandfather, along with millions of others, was infected with tuberculosis. He spent a year in a sanitorium in Arizona. Thankfully, he recovered. Many did not.

Once medical researchers developed a tuberculosis vaccine, a new "killer" emerged—cancer. Later in the century, AIDS became the new, feared epidemic, sweeping across Africa and into the rest of the world.

Vaccinations offer us some control over the spread of disease; they do not, however, control the evolution of new diseases.

That ability to control disease carries a heady responsibility. Why were the diseases present in the first place? Were there any hidden, unexpected gifts in contracting and then recovering from these illnesses?

When I was a child, my brother, sister and I all contracted and then recovered from measles, chicken pox and mumps. Thankfully, none of us had any side effects. In that era, a small percentage of children had permanent damage from the illnesses, e.g., sterility and deafness.

Research shows that these relatively mild illnesses actually benefit the body. After a fever, children usually experience a spurt in emotional maturation. The immune system also develops and strengthens as it responds to viral infections.

When the Clintons developed their "health plan," one of the cornerstones of their policy was childhood vaccinations. The policy clearly stated that the purpose of the vaccines was to benefit the *parents*, not the children. The vaccines were intended to save the adults lost days at work—the "inconvenience" of staying home to nurse a sick child.

The Downside of Vaccines

While vaccines clearly offer many benefits, we are also beginning to see the potential pitfalls in administering them. Short-term effects include fever, malaise, joint and muscle pain and general flu-like symptoms. Most vaccine reaction studies track children for only *five days* after receiving a vaccination. Long-term side effects are more severe, including autism (one of the main severe side effects of the MMR vaccine), altered brain development, seizures, loss of brain synapses (nerve cell connections), and permanent brain damage.

Very few doctors counsel their patients about the potential side effects of vaccines. The epidemiologists, who study epidemic diseases, are not focused on the outcome for individual patients. They study the effect on entire populations, with an understanding that any mass application of medicine will cause "collateral damage." That sterile, scientific term is rather meaningless, unless the "collateral damage" includes one or more of your children.

Physicians in the U.S. are supposed to report the side effects of vaccine administration. CDC acknowledges, however, that vaccine reactions are underreported. Each year the CDC receives more than 30,000 reports of adverse reactions to vaccines. Ten-to-15 percent of the vaccine reactions are classified as serious (resulting in permanent disability, hospitalization, life-threatening illnesses or death). Considering this is a voluntary system, the exact number of children who react is likely many times higher.

Only now are the children of the first great wave of vaccinations reaching their later, mature years. Now we are also learning that certain vaccines do not last for an entire lifetime. Those who received vaccinations as children may be vulnerable to diseases they assume they are immune to, e.g., smallpox, tetanus and chicken pox.

How to decide?

With my own children, I weighed the benefits and the side effects to decide whether to have any vaccines and, if yes, which ones and the best administration schedule to follow.

The best of all possible worlds is to be an unvaccinated person in a vaccinated population. That means you don't expose yourself or your children to the vaccine and you are very unlikely to be exposed to the disease.

Traveling to a country where few people are vaccinated would mean your child is unvaccinated in an environment where they are VERY likely to encounter diseases. This is the worst case scenario: being an unvaccinated person in an unvaccinated population.

Keep in mind that you can pick and choose which vaccines you want your child to receive. Many parents take an "all-or-nothing" stance. Although this is an inexact guessing game, with no fool-proof crystal ball to read the future, I would encourage you to consider the following factors:

- Am I willing to live with the possibility that my child may react to a vaccine?
- Am I able and willing to stay at home with my child if she is unvaccinated and develops an illness? Pertussis (whooping cough), for example, may require six weeks or more of convalescence before complete recovery.
- Will my child be traveling in the future? Where? Outside the U.S.?
- How is my child's overall health? Is his immune system strong?
- What am I doing to support my child's health overall?
- What activities may increase my child's exposure to a disease or infection, e.g., child care, living in a rural area, or living in a crowded urban environment?

For my own sons, I chose to have them vaccinated for tetanus. I opted for this vaccine because we live in a rural area where the boys commonly encounter sharp, rusty, metal objects. Tetanus is one of the "cleanest" of the vaccines, meaning that it has few side effects. The challenge with tetanus, however, is to find a source for the vaccine that does not also include pertussis, which is one of the "dirtiest" vaccines, meaning it causes a great number of side effects.

How to minimize side effects of vaccines

If you choose to vaccinate, *wait as long as possible to administer the vaccines.* Ideally, your child would be at least four years old, when the immune system is more fully developed. Conventional doctors say very early vaccinations are better, precisely because the immune system is NOT fully developed and the body can not react as much to the vaccine. Classical Medicine suggests the opposite: Instead of overwhelming an incompletely developed immune system, wait to expose the child to vaccine when the immune system is more fully developed.

Hilary Andrews, N.D. has deeply researched the effects of vaccinations on both adults and young children. Her investigations revealed that the schedule developed by the U.S. Advisory Committee on Immunization Practices (ACIP) for administering vaccines was based primarily on convenience. Conventional physicians see children more in their first 3 – 5 years than at any other time in their life. The schedule was NOT developed to accommodate children's developing immune systems, but rather for the convenience of pediatricians administering the vaccines.

Administer one vaccine at a time. The vaccine cited with causing the greatest number of reactions, particularly autism, is the MMRV (measles, mumps, rubella, varicella/chicken pox) vaccine. Until recently, pediatricians usually gave the MMR vaccine (already one of the "dirtiest" combination vaccines) separately from the chicken pox vaccination. The first dose of the MMRV vaccine is associated with rash and higher rates of fever than MMR and varicella vaccines given separately. One in 20 people have a rash, while 1 in 5 have a fever. Seizures caused by high fever five-to-12 days after the first dose are more common with the MMRV vaccine than with the MMR.

If you choose to give your child these vaccines, discuss with your pediatrician the possibility of administering these vaccines separately, spaced at least one month apart. Depending on the vaccine manufacturers, sometimes this is difficult if not impossible to do. When I chose to have the boys vaccinated with tetanus, I was unable to find a source of tetanus-only vaccine.

Choose vaccines that do NOT contain Thimerosal (mercury) or aluminum. Although the ACIP had conclusive evidence that thimerosal contributed to autism and other brain injuries, they did not ban the use of mercury in vaccines until November 2002. Vaccines still contain traces of thimerosal because the mercury-containing compound is added to vaccines to preserve them; then, the mercury is exposed to chelates to remove the heavy metal. Small traces of mercury, however, still remain in the vaccines.

Vaccines also contain aluminum which is toxic to the nervous system, contributing to both learning and behavioral deficits. Manufacturers add aluminum to vaccines to trigger the T-helper cell 2 (Th2)-mediated cell response, driving production of Immune globulin E (IgE) which is associated with anaphylactic allergies. Ideally, during the first year of life an infant's immune system would be directed toward T-helper cell 1 (Th1) cell responses, which develop the baby's ability to respond to acute infections. "Goosing" the infant's body with vaccines to mobilize the Th2 response increases the development of allergies and auto-immune conditions.

Proponents of vaccinations argue that mothers' milk naturally delivers small amounts of aluminum, about 2.0 micrograms (mcgs). In contrast, infants receiving the complete recommended schedule of vaccinations were exposed to 225 to 1750 mcgs of aluminum. This is an extremely high exposure even for an adult. A high dose impacts the tiny body of an infant even more strongly. According to Dr. Hilary Andrews, we also have no research on the effects of *injecting* aluminum, which is a completely different delivery route than aluminum absorbed through the digestive tract, such as in mother's milk. We do not know if injected aluminum is stored in body tissues or properly excreted from the body.

Minimize extra activities after the vaccination. This allows your child to rest during a time her immune system will be working very hard to respond to the vaccine. In addition, if she does react to the vaccine, you will have fewer confounding factors to cloud an assessment of what caused the reaction (e.g., was it the vaccine, or the chlorine at the pool?).

Vaccine reactions

If your child does react to a vaccine, certain homeopathic remedies can help moderate the side effects of vaccines. Contact your naturopathic physician or classical homeopath for instructions about which homeopathic remedy would be best for your child.

Most vaccine research only tracks vaccine reactions that occur within 5 – 14 days of the administration of a vaccine. The neurological and behavioral changes associated with vaccinations, however, may take years to fully manifest.

If you believe your child has reacted to a vaccine, contact your family physician. Your family doctor may or may not report this information to the Center for Disease Control (CDC). Remember, physicians are *not* required to report vaccine reactions.

Either you or your physician can file a Vaccine Adverse Event Reporting System (VAERS) Form by visiting the VAERS website at www.vaers.hhs.gov, or by calling 1-800-822-7967.

In addition, you can contact The National Vaccine Injury Compensation Program. The very fact that this agency exists speaks volumes. The federal government created this program to help people who may have been harmed by a vaccine. For details about the National Vaccine Injury Compensation Program, call 1-800-338-2382 or visit their Web site at *www.hrsa.gov/vaccinecompensation.*

Alternatives to vaccination

Indian homeopaths have a track record of using homeopathic remedies to replace conventional vaccines. Homeopathy is widely practiced in India, in part because the medicines are inexpensive and easy to administer. In addition, India has a long history of choosing natural medicines.

In the Bengal Allen Medical Institute, physicians have developed a homeopathic immunization schedule, beginning when the child is three months old.

CAUTION: You will need the help of a trained homeopath to guide you in taking these homeopathic medicines.

3-to-9 months

- Tuberculinum bovinum homeopathic remedy in place of Bacille Calmette-Guérin (BCG) vaccine for tuberculosis
- Diphtherium, Pertussin and then Tetanotoxin (at an interval of 1-to-2 months between each remedy) in place of the diphtheria, pertussis and tetanus (DPT) vaccine
- Lathyrus sativus homeopathic remedy in place of oral polio vaccine (OPV)

9-to-12 months

- Morbillium homeopathic remedy (measles)

18-to-24 months

- Diphtherium, Pertussin and then Tetanotoxin (at an interval of 1-to-2 months between each remedy) in place of the diphtheria, pertussis and tetanus (DPT) booster dose
- Lathyrus sativus in place of the OPV booster dose

5-to-6 years

- Diphtherinum, then Tetanotoxin, in place of the diphtheria-tetanus (DT) booster dose
- Baptisia homeopathic remedy in place of typhoid vaccine (usually not a common concern in North America; a major concern in India and most of Asia).

10 years

- Tetanotoxin homeopathic remedy, in place of tetanus booster shot

Subrata Kamar Banerjea, M.D.(H), a renowned homeopathic physician and medical author, notes a very low success rate with Lathyrus sativus (for preventing polio) and Diptherium (for preventing diphtheria). He reports much higher success rates with Tuberculinum (tuberculosis), Baptisia (typhoid) and Pertussis (whooping cough).

In this country, testing homeopathic vaccines raises ethical questions—what if children receiving the experimental homeopathic remedies contract the disease? Research to date on homeopathic vaccinations does *not* demonstrate an increase in antibodies to the disease. How, then, is the body responding to the remedies and preventing disease? Some homeopaths suggest the body responds on a "deeper" level than antibody formation.

Some homeopaths suggest using homeopathic vaccines only during epidemic outbreaks of diseases, for short-term prevention.

In general, homeopaths do NOT recommend taking homeopathic remedies unless they are needed. This homeopathic vaccination protocol is outside the realm of "classical" homeopathy. Usually a homeopath would wait until a child developed symptoms. Only then would the homeopath prescribe a remedy to address that patient's particular set of symptoms.

Another option is to expose your children to some of these early childhood illnesses on purpose. In the 1950's, teen-aged girls had Rubella "parties." When a girl came down with German measles, she invited her friends over to play, hoping to spread the disease to them. Young women wanted to have this illness before becoming pregnant, to avoid the potentially damaging effects of the disease on a developing fetus.

I've tried, so far unsuccessfully, to expose my boys to chicken pox. I would prefer them to develop natural resistance to the infection, rather than having the vaccine.

What to tell the school

In most states, parents are required to show proof that their children have been vaccinated. In Colorado, I am allowed to declare that I have chosen not to vaccinate for religious reasons. At this time, health choices are not considered a valid reason for bypassing the vaccination process.

Childhood diseases

Remember that you may choose to have some, but not all, of the vaccines. See the list below of childhood illnesses; the natural course of the disease and its potential consequences; and reported side effects of the vaccine.

Measles (Rubeola; Morbilli; 9-day measles)

Incubation: 8-to-21 days
Infectious: Four days before and 5-to-10 days after rash appears
Spread: by respiratory droplets, or contact with objects infected with nasal/oral secretions.

Measles is a highly contagious viral infection that commonly affects children. Measles usually begin with two-to-four days of fever, runny nose and hacking cough, followed by the appearance of Koplik's spots (white spots, like a grain of white sand surrounded by a red ring) that appear on the insides of the cheeks and lips. Skin rash usually appears three-to-five days after symptoms begin. Other bacterial infections, such as pneumonia or ear infection, can accompany the measles.

Globally, measles infect about 30-to-40 million people every year; around 800,000 die. Malnourished children, especially those with vitamin A deficiency, are most likely to die from the disease. Children in developed countries, with good nutrition, rarely have complications from measles. In the U.S., where vaccination is common, about 100-to-300 people develop measles each year.

Possible complication: blindness, usually in malnourished, vitamin A-deficient children. Other possible complications include ear infection, pneumonia, seizures (jerking and staring), brain damage and death.

Immunity: Mothers who have had the measles transfer immunity to the fetus, protecting the baby through the first year of life. Having the measles gives lifelong immunity.

Mumps

Incubation: 12-to-28 days
Infectious: two days before salivary glands swell until after the swelling resolves
Spread: by respiratory droplets and direct contact with the saliva of an infected person. Usually a mild childhood infection, mumps causes fever, headache, swelling of the salivary glands in the cheeks and sometimes swelling under the tongue and jaw.

Complications: mumps can cause deafness, meningitis (infection of the brain and spinal cord covering), painful swelling of the testicles or ovaries and, rarely, death.

Rubella (German Measles)

Incubation: 14-to-23 days
Infectious: five days before and seven days after rash appears
Spread: by nasal and throat secretions and respiratory droplets. Infected infants can spread the virus via throat secretions and/or urine. Rubella usually is a short-lived infection, beginning with a rash behind the ears or on the face that spreads down the body. The virus can also cause mild fever, watery eyes, lymph node swelling and joint pain (mostly in women).
Complications: If a woman contracts rubella while she is pregnant, she could have a miscarriage or give birth to a baby with serious birth defects. Before the rubella vaccine was developed, infected girls would have "rubella parties," inviting other girls so they would have the infection and develop immunity before becoming pregnant.

Reactions to the measles, mumps, rubella (MMR) vaccine

Mild Problems

- Fever (up to 1 out of 6 people)
- Mild rash (about 1 out of 20)
- Swelling of glands in the cheeks or neck (rare)

These problems usually occur 7-to-12 days after the shot. They are less common after the second dose.

Moderate Problems

- Seizure (jerking or staring) caused by fever (about 1 out of 3,000 doses)
- Temporary pain and stiffness in the joints, mostly in teenage or adult women (up to 1 out of 4)
- Temporary low platelet count, which can cause a bleeding disorder (about 1 out of 30,000 doses)

Severe Problems (Very Rare)

- Serious allergic reaction (less than 1 out of a million doses)

- Deafness
- Long-term seizures, coma or lowered consciousness
- Permanent brain damage

Remember that MMRV (measles, mumps, rubella and chicken pox) vaccines cause even more reactions, with increased reports of fevers and rashes, usually occurring five-to-12 days after the first dose of the vaccine.

Tuberculosis

Incubation: four-to-12 weeks from exposure to positive tuberculosis test.
Infectious: respiratory droplets spread by coughing, singing and/or strong exhalation. Initially tuberculosis usually goes unnoticed, with complete healing of lesions. Ninety-to-95 percent of those infected have no after-effects, other than occasional lymph node calcification in the lung and bronchial areas. Approximately five-to-10 percent of those infected progress to pulmonary tuberculosis, usually within one-to-two years after the primary infection. Common symptoms include a productive cough, bloody sputum, chest pain and shortness of breath. Rarely tuberculosis spreads to other organs, e.g., the kidneys, bones, skin and intestines.

Diphtheria

Incubation: two-to-5 days
Infectious: varies, depending on how long the bacteria remain in the infected person's secretions—usually 2-to-4 weeks.
Spread: by contact with an infected person; infected raw, unpasteurized milk.
Diphtheria usually affects children under 15 years of age and causes a thick covering in the back of the throat that can lead to breathing problems, paralysis, heart failure and even death. Immunity to diphtheria declines over time, whether that immunity was developed by exposure to the disease or vaccination.

Tetanus (Lockjaw)

Incubation: usually three-to-21 days, but in some cases may range to several months, depending on the extent and location of the wound.
Infectious: soil, or fomites, contaminated with human or other animal feces.
Spread: into puncture or open wounds infected with soil, street dust, human or other animal feces. Occasionally tetanus passes via intravenous street drugs or surgical procedures. Tetanus causes painful tightening of the muscles, usually all over the body. Tetanus can lead to "locking" of the jaw, so that the child cannot swallow or open her mouth. Tetanus leads to death in up to 2 out of 10 cases.

Pertussis (Whooping Cough)

Incubation: seven-to-21 days
Infectious: up to 3-to-4 weeks after the illness begins
Spreads: by respiratory droplets.

Whooping cough begins with a slight fever and runny nose, which develops into a loose cough. Within one-to-two weeks the mucous thickens, making it difficult to expectorate, triggering violent coughing spells ending with a high-pitched "whoop" that can last for six-to-10 weeks. Infants with whooping cough may have a hard time eating, drinking and/or breathing.

Complications: Whooping cough can lead to pneumonia, seizures (jerking and staring spells), brain damage and death. Ninety percent of deaths are in children under one year of age and 75 percent are under six months of age.

Reactions to the diphtheria, tetanus, pertussis (DTaP) vaccine

Mild Problems (Common)

- Fever (1 in 4 children)
- Redness or swelling where the shot was given (1 child in 4)
- Soreness or tenderness where the shot was given (1 child in 4)

These problems occur more often after the fourth and fifth doses of the DTaP series than after earlier doses. Sometimes, after the fourth or fifth dose of DTaP vaccine, the entire arm or leg in which the shot was given swells, lasting one to seven days (1 child in 30).

Other mild problems include

- Fussiness (1 child in 3)
- Tiredness or poor appetite (1 child in 10)
- Vomiting (1 child in 50)

These problems generally occur one to three days after the shot.

Moderate Problems (Uncommon)

- Seizure (jerking or staring) (1 child out of 14,000)
- Non-stop crying, for three hours or more (1 child out of 1,000)
- High fever, over 105°F (1 child out of 16,000)

Severe Problems (Very Rare)

- Serious allergic reaction (less than 1 out of a million doses)
- Long-term seizures, coma or lowered consciousness
- Permanent brain damage

Poliomyelitis

Incubation: usually seven-to-14 days but up to 35 days

Infectious: not accurately known. Virus persists in the throat secretions for about a week and up to six weeks in the feces.

Spread: by nasal and throat secretions; oral-fecal transmission (e.g., through water or food contaminated with feces).

Polio is an acute viral illness that can cause a range of symptoms, from mild fever, fatigue, headache, nausea and vomiting to severe paralysis. The site of paralysis depends on where nerve cells in the brain or spinal cord are damaged. Usually the paralysis is asymmetrical, effecting one side more than the other. About 1 in 100 people who contract polio progress to muscle paralysis. About two out of three of those who develop paralysis have permanent weakness.

Polio vaccine

Some pediatricians in the United States do not administer polio vaccine as cases of Poliomyelitis are increasingly rare in this country. In four countries, however, polio is still endemic: Nigeria, India, Pakistan and Afghanistan. Sometimes the "wild" virus in these regions is carried to previously polio-free regions.

Most cases of polio in the United States result from vaccination with the Oral Polio Vaccine (OPV).

Herpes varicella-zoster (Chicken pox):

Incubation: usually 11-to 15 days, but can be up to three weeks.

Infectious: one-to-two days before the rash develops, until five days after the rash resolves.

Spreads: by direct contact with skin lesions, respiratory droplets, or contact with contaminated objects.

Chicken pox is an acute viral disease with sudden onset of low-grade fever, fatigue and rash. Chicken pox usually affects children. Rarely is the disease fatal. The skin is covered with itchy, honey-colored vesicles that crust over and heal within three-to-four days. These lesions may appear on the skin, particularly areas irritated by sunburn or diaper rash; the scalp; the mouth; the respiratory tract; and/or around the eyes.

Complications: The symptoms can be much more severe in adults, newborns up to 10 days old and immune compromised adults and children.

Reactions to the chicken pox vaccine

Mild Problems

- Soreness or swelling where the shot was given (about 1 out of 5 children and up to 1 out of 3 adolescents and adults)
- Fever (1 out of 10 people)
- Mild rash, up to a month after vaccination (1 person out of 25). Rarely, these people infect other members of their household with chicken pox.

Moderate Problems

- Seizure (jerking or staring) caused by fever (very rare).

Severe Problems

- Pneumonia (very rare)
- Other serious problems, including severe brain reactions and low blood count, have been reported after chickenpox vaccination.

Note: The first dose of MMRV vaccine has been associated with rash and higher rates of fever than MMR and varicella vaccines given separately. Rash has been reported in about one person in 20 and fever in about one person in five. Seizures caused by a fever are also reported more often after MMRV. These usually occur five to 12 days after the first dose.

CHAPTER 6

For Adults Only

This chapter offers special guidance for adults and their special needs. Here you will find information about soothing nausea in pregnancy, quelling menstrual cramps and addressing prostatitis. You will also find frank discussions on supporting longevity, e.g., optimizing bone health and enhancing libido.

BONE HEALTH

The best time to build bone is before age 35, when we reach peak bone mineral density. Men naturally have more bone than women, in part because of their taller, larger skeletons. Men also have relatively higher testosterone levels, the primary hormone that stimulates the osteoblasts—cells that lay down new bone.

The bones must be stressed in order to catalyze them to lay down new bone. By "stressed," I do not mean "break" the bone. Instead, the bone must be traumatized on a micro-level for the bone to get the message to rebuild.

Exercise is the primary healthy "stressor" that signals the development of new bone. Every time you contract a muscle, the tendon pulls against the bone and traumatizes the bone on a cellular level. This micro-trauma stimulates new bone development.

In addition, the bone is a crystalline structure. We know from crystal research, the foundation of much of the computer industry, as well as the early radio technology, that compressing a crystal generates an electromagnetic charge. When your bones are compressed, e.g., with the weight of walking, the bones develop a "Piezo-electric effect." A tiny current of electricity passes through the crystalline structure of the bone, which also catalyzes re-mineralization.

The more we exercise as children and teenagers, the more bone density we will lay down. The better we eat during these formative years, the greater the bone density we will build as well.

Foods naturally rich in calcium and other minerals top the list of bone-healthy foods. Leafy green vegetables are rich in calcium. The plant structure releases calcium much more easily than protein-bound animal forms of calcium. A cup of cow's milk, for example, contains about 300 mg of calcium. Only about 100 mg—*less than one-third* of that calcium, however—is easily absorbed. In contrast, about 67 percent of the calcium in kale is easily absorbed and over 65 percent of the calcium in cabbage is well-absorbed. Eating a cup of kale delivers roughly the same amount of *absorbable* calcium as a cup of cow's milk.

Bone bombs

I call colas "bone bombs" because they deliver several bone-destroying foods in one neat package: sugar, caffeine and phosphorus.

Sugar acidifies the body, as do other simple carbohydrates. The more of the "white wonders" (white sugar, white flour and white rice) you eat, the more acidic the body becomes. The body pulls calcium from the bones to buffer this acidity and return the body to normal pH.

Caffeine also acidifies the body, thereby increasing calcium loss.

Phosphorus competes with calcium for uptake across the intestines and into the bloodstream. When levels are high enough, phosphorus begins to replace calcium in the bones, creating a weaker, more brittle bone. The same process happens when we take bisphosphonates, such as Fosamax (alendronate sodium). These pharmaceutical drugs do increase bone density. What the bone mineral density test cannot reveal, however, is how much of that mineral is calcium and how much is phosphorus, which produces the weaker, more brittle bone.

Studies have demonstrated that the more sweetened cola drinks teenagers consume, the lower their bone mineral density later in life. As a teenager you are setting the stage for lifelong bone health.

Exercise during the teens and twenties also dramatically influences bone mineralization. The more a person is able to exercise, the greater her bone density will be at age 35-to-40.

An additive approach to bone health

1   Diet and exercise
2   Supplements

3   Bio-identical hormones
4   Bisphosphonates

I place both diet and exercise as Number 1, because both are equally important in building and maintaining strong bone. Your diet provides the building blocks for healthy bone; exercise signals the bone to use these nutrients to construct or repair bone.

Diet

Most dietary recommendations focus on increasing calcium to improve bone density. Calcium alone, however, cannot build strong bones. Imagine walking into a symphony hall to hear a performance of Beethoven's Ninth Symphony. When the curtain goes up, only one clarinetist is sitting on the stage.

Expecting calcium alone to build strong bone is like expecting the clarinetist to play the entire symphony. The clarinetist is important, but she can't play all of the parts. Similarly, calcium is an important player in building bone, but calcium alone cannot build strong bone. In fact, if you supplement high amounts of calcium without the balance of other nutrients, the body will begin to deposit calcium in joint capsules and muscle tissue. Without the other nutrients, the body cannot utilize these high levels of calcium.

Our bones are composed of two major components: osteocalcin and minerals. Osteocalcin is a flexible, spongy connective tissue matrix. Minerals are embedded into osteocalcin. Studies of traditional South African women have demonstrated that these women have low bone mineral density, yet they also have low fracture rates. The working hypothesis is that they have healthy, flexible osteocalcin that absorbs physical shocks and traumas without fracturing.

We currently do not have any tests to check the health and flexibility of osteocalcin. All we have are machines that test the amount of mineral packed into the bone (bone mineral density scans). While the amount of bone density if vitally important, the tests only tell half the story.

If all we have is a hammer (the bone mineral density test), then everything looks like a nail. In other words, if we only have machines that test bone density, we will focus on bone density as the most important factor for bone health.

Bone density is a vital component of bone health, but bone mineralization alone does not tell the entire story. Nutrients that support healthy connective tissue development, e.g., vitamin C and zinc, may be at least as important to bone health as calcium, even though we cannot "prove" their effect on osteocalcin and, thus, bone health.

Acid/alkaline balance and bone health

The more acid-forming foods you eat, the more calcium the body pulls from the bone to buffer the increased acidity. Acid-forming foods include many people's favorite foods: meat, eggs, dairy, sugar, alcohol and coffee.

A study conducted in *1920* demonstrated that people who ate plant sources of protein lost one-third *less* calcium than those who ate animal protein. The more meat, milk and eggs you eat, the more calcium you lose. The more plant sources of protein you eat, the more calcium stays in your bones.

Calcium loss effects bone density more dramatically than calcium intake or calcium absorption. In other words, the amount of calcium we *lose* impacts bone health more dramatically than the amount of calcium we *absorb*. A high-protein diet increases uric acid formation, which taxes our bones as well as our kidneys.

Animal and plant proteins have different effects on the body. Animal proteins have more sulfur-containing amino acids, which increase acidity in the body. Methionine, a sulfur-containing amino acid particularly high in meats, eggs and dairy products, is converted to homocysteine. Elevated homocysteine levels may increase bone loss. Plant proteins, in contrast, contain a very small percentage of these sulfur-containing amino acids and do not have the same acidifying effect in the body.

Easy to absorb forms of calcium

Despite what the American Daily Council tells us, many humans do not digest cow's milk well. On a global scale, most of us can digest milk only until age two or three, and human milk is the milk of choice. For a listing of lactose intolerance by populations, see Chapter 5.

Each animal's milk stimulates different types of growth. Human milk, for instance, is high in essential fatty acids and stimulates brain and neural development. In contrast, a baby calf's first priority is to stand and walk, so cow's milk stimulates muscle development.

Animal sources of calcium are also much more difficult for your body to assimilate than plant sources, as you can see from the following chart. Although lower in calcium, plant sources are easier for your body to absorb. One cup of Chinese cabbage, for example, delivers almost as much calcium as a cup of milk.

Food Source Calcium Content (mg) % Absorbed Calcium Absorbed

Beans, pinto (1/2 cup)	44.7 mg of calcium	17% absorbed	7.6 mg absorbable calcium
Broccoli (1/2 cup)	35 mg of calcium	53% absorbed	18.4 mg absorbable calcium
Brussels sprouts (1/2 cup)	19 mg of calcium	64% absorbed	12 mg absorbable calcium
Cabbage, Chinese (1 cup)	158 mg calcium	54% absorbed	86 mg absorbable calcium
Cabbage, Green (1 cup)	50 mg of calcium	65% absorbed	32 mg absorbable calcium
Kale (1 cup)	94 mg calcium	59% absorbed	56 mg absorbable calcium
Mustard greens (1 cup)	94 mg calcium	58% absorbed	74 mg absorbable calcium
Sesame seeds (1 ounce)	28 mg calcium	21% absorbed	7.7 mg of absorbable calcium
Tofu, raw, firm (1/2 cup)	258 mg calcium	31% absorbed	80 mg absorbable calcium
Turnip greens (1 cup)	198 mg calcium	52% absorbed	102 mg absorbable calcium
Cow's milk (1 cup)	300 mg calcium	32% absorbed	96 mg absorbable calcium

Note: One cup of Chinese cabbage contains roughly the same amount of absorbable calcium as a cup of cow's milk.

Calcium supplements

If you are concerned about bone health, your physician may advise you to take an antacid that contains calcium carbonate (e.g., Tums™). Unfortunately antacids are poor sources of calcium for two reasons:

- Calcium and all minerals need an acidic environment in the stomach to break down. Antacids by their very nature reduce stomach acidity. Elderly people often have more difficulty absorbing minerals and other nutrients because they produce less stomach acid. About 40 percent of postmenopausal women are severely deficient in stomach acid. You can maximize absorption by taking mineral supplements with an acidic fruit juice (e.g., grapefruit juice) or food.

- Calcium carbonate, made from seashells, is difficult for the digestive tract to break down and absorb. "Chelated" forms of minerals—i.e., a mineral attached to an amino acid—are easier for the stomach to break down than minerals bound to other minerals. Examples of calcium chelates include calcium citrate, calcium malate and calcium aspartate.
- See below for more information about how to maximize the benefit of all your supplements.

How much calcium do I need?

The amount of calcium you need depends on your diet and the amount and variety of other nutrients you are supplementing. Recent research suggests taking too much calcium by itself can actually increase risk of hip fracture. Remember that in order for calcium to be absorbed and properly used in the body, ALL of the other nutrients must be present.

Postmenopausal women need approximately 1,000 mg of calcium a day. If you are supplementing calcium citrate or malate, you can reduce that amount by one-quarter to one-half because these calcium supplements are more easily absorbed than calcium carbonate.

What About the Ratio of Calcium to Magnesium?

We do not have a definitive answer about the best ratio of calcium to magnesium. Some studies suggest taking twice as much calcium as magnesium, others advocate equal amounts and still others recommend twice as much magnesium as calcium. I recommend you supplement at least half as much magnesium as calcium. If you are taking 600 mg of calcium citrate, for example, you should take at least 300 mg of magnesium.

What other supplements support bone health?

Vitamin D

This vital bone building nutrient increases calcium absorption in the intestines and deposition in the bones. When exposed to sunlight, cholesterol in our skin converts to vitamin D. Even 20 minutes of sun exposure in northern climates should be enough to generate sufficient quantities of vitamin D. Fish, eggs and liver also contain significant amounts. Vegetarians who get little sun exposure may need to supplement vitamin D. Recommended amounts: 1,000 IU. daily.

NOTE: Recent research on the benefits of vitamin D have led physicians and nutritionists to recommend astronomically higher doses of vitamin D. Unless someone suffers with a medical condition associated with low vitamin D levels (e.g., M.S.), I don't recommend extremely high doses of vitamin D. These mega-dose recommendations are based on the "take-this-for-that" mentality of viewing nutrients in isolation. A high dose of any one nutrient will cause an imbalance in other nutrient levels, because different nutrients compete for uptake. Extremely high doses of vitamin D, for example, will cause a reduction in other fat soluble nutrients in the body, e.g., vitamins A, E and K. I have one post-menopausal M.S. patient, for example, who had a return of menstrual bleeding when her vitamin D levels were too high. Vitamin D had artificially driven down vitamin K levels, a nutrient vital for normal blood clotting. When her body could not maintain normal blood clotting factors, she began to bleed.

Vitamin C

In addition to numerous other functions, vitamin C promotes the normal formation and cross-linking of proteins that make up part of our bones' structure. Recommended amounts: at least 1,000 mg per day, divided into three or more doses. When taking more than 1,000 mg per day, be sure to take *buffered* Vitamin C, to avoid acidifying the body too much.

Manganese

Manganese encourages the production of protein-like molecules called mucopolysaccharides. These saccharides form a base for calcium deposits in the bones. Without manganese, the body cannot pack calcium into the bones. Recommended amounts: 15-to-30 mg per day.

Boron

Boron is an important co-factor for the synthesis of testosterone and 17 beta-estradiol. In addition, supplementing boron reduces urinary loss of calcium and magnesium by 44 percent. Recommended amounts: 3 mg per day.

B6, B12 and folic acid

As mentioned above, high animal protein intake can result in the formation of more homocysteine, an amino acid that has been linked with increased risk for osteoporosis and heart disease. Homocysteine normally converts to other less harmful byproducts if the body has adequate amounts of three important nutrients: B6, B12 and folic acid. Recommended amounts: 50-to-100 mg of B6, 400-800 mcg folic acid and 3-15 mcg of B12.

Zinc

Important for many functions in the body, zinc enhances the activity of vitamin D. Zinc promotes the normal synthesis of DNA and protein, making it a vital nutrient for the formation of proteins in the bone, osteoblasts (bone builders) and osteoclasts (bone destroyers). Recommended amounts: 15-to-30 mg per day.

Strontium

A study in Canada demonstrated that non-radioactive strontium increased bone density in patients who had bone cancer. Anyone who has known or worked with someone with bone cancer knows this is a miraculous response! Strontium also stimulates bone building activity in healthy bone. Recommended amount: 2 mg daily.

Gemmotherapy botanicals

Gemmotherapies are herbal supplements prepared from the buds and new shoots of plants, primarily trees. Several gemmotherapy remedies help support bone mineralization. Ideally, you would work with a health care provider trained in gemmotherapy remedies to help you select the most appropriate medicines for your particular health care needs.

How to Maximize Supplement Absorption

- Choose encapsulated or gel-cap supplements. Tablets can be very difficult for the stomach to break down, particularly mineral tablets. Digesting a hard-packed mineral tablet is a bit like trying to break down a pebble. The tablet may pass through the digestive tract unchanged.
- To determine whether your *mineral* tablet will break down: Drop one mineral tablet in six ounces of room-temperature vinegar and stir every two to three minutes. After 30 minutes the mineral tablet should have disintegrated into small particles. If the tablet has not broken down, do not use that supplement.

- Choose a good multivitamin and mineral supplement rather than a handful of single nutrients. The nutrients function best together, not in isolation.
- The Recommended Daily Allowance (RDA) aims to prevent major diseases, not promote optimal health. Each body has different nutritional requirements. Ask a health care provider trained in nutrition what amounts of nutrients are optimal for you.
- Choose a multivitamin and mineral that requires four-to-six capsules per day. You cannot squeeze an adequate amount of nutrients into a single multivitamin and mineral tablet or capsule.
- Avoid supplements that contain dyes and preservatives.
- If you have food allergies, read labels carefully. Many supplement manufacturers now list common food allergens, e.g., corn, dairy, yeast and wheat.

Exercise

In order to encourage mineral uptake, you need at least three hours per week of weight-bearing exercise. "Weight-bearing" does NOT mean weightlifting. Weight bearing refers to exercise that requires us to carry weight with the spine and "long bones" —the femur in the thigh and the fibula and tibia in the lower legs.

Weightlifting also can help with bone density, as can any exercise that causes a strong muscle contraction. When a muscle contracts, its tendon pulls against the bone, which slightly traumatizes the bone in that area. This "microtrauma" signals the bone to take up minerals and repair this section of bone. If the bones are never traumatized, they never get the message to repair and rejuvenate.

Although weight-bearing exercise is best, even non-weight-bearing exercise benefits the bone. Swimming increases bone mineral density, as does stretching and tai chi. Any movement will benefit the bone. Be sure to choose movements that your bones can support.

After one of my friends received news that she had osteoporosis, she decided to start jump-roping. The next day, the middle of her back was in severe pain, right in the spinal area. She tried several different ways of addressing the pain. After several recommendations that she have a spinal X-ray, she finally consented. The X-ray revealed that she had fractured one of her thoracic vertebrae. If she had gone earlier for testing, she might have been a candidate for the newer bone repair surgery—balloon kyphoplasty. During this procedure, the surgeon inserts and then inflates two small balloons in the collapsed spinal bone and then injects special cement into the bones to repair the fracture. Unfortunately, my friend was beyond the two-month recommended period before she was diagnosed.

The message here is that vigorous, pounding exercise is a great way to build bone during our teens and twenties and possibly into our thirties. After that time, though, when we are rebuilding bone, heavy impact exercise can damage instead of support bone. *Choose exercise that will stress but not fracture the bone. Initially, aim for too gentle rather than too vigorous exercise, particularly if you have been diagnosed with osteoporosis.*

Bio-identical hormones

Our bones are like buildings that are constantly being demolished and rebuilt. The better we eat and the more we exercise as children and young adults, the bigger the "house" we build. Bone-building cells are called "osteoblasts," and bone-demolishing cells are called "osteoclasts."

After age 40, the bone demolition crew starts to outrun the construction crew and we begin to lose bone. The demolition crew really speeds up during the first two-to-five years of menopause.

Estrogen blocks the activity of the osteoclasts, thereby helping to *maintain* bone density. Testosterone increases the activity of osteoblasts, the cells that lay down new bone. Progesterone may have some effect on increasing osteoblast activity.

I only prescribe bio-identical hormones for women who are not able to maintain or build bone with diet, exercise and supplements. Usually, we follow a treatment plan utilizing these lifestyle choices and supplements for a year and then retest bone density. We follow the plan for a year because bone is slow-moving tissue that takes time to respond to treatment. Repeating the bone mineral density scan in a year helps the patient and I evaluate whether they are on target or need to do more to support bone density. The next step after diet, exercise and nutritional supplements is to add bio-identical hormones.

Work with a health care provider who understands the functions of bio-identical hormones (the ones that exactly duplicate the hormones our body makes) and can prescribe the "friendliest" forms of hormone replacement therapy.

Remember that even bio-identical hormones potentially can cause side effects. Some patients think that bio-identical hormones are perfectly harmless because they are more "natural." Like fire, these hormones can heal or burn. Use hormones, or any supplement, with respect. Take only as much as you need (more definitely is *not* better when it comes to hormones), for as long as you need them.

If you decide to stop taking estrogen, be sure to wean off *slowly*, usually over six to 12 months. This slow withdrawal is similar to the slow drop in hormones during peri-menopause. Usually, the most severe, debilitating menopausal symptoms occur after sudden, precipitous drops in hormone levels. After removing the ovaries, for example, reproductive hormone levels drop to post-menopausal levels within 24 hours. When the body makes this transition naturally, that hormonal drop usually will occur over six months to 10 years!

Bisphosphonates

These pharmaceutical drugs have two primary functions: They block the activity of the osteoclasts—cells that break down bone—and they pack phosphorus instead of calcium into the bone. Bone mineral density will increase, usually over a three-month period. What the bone mineral density scan cannot show, however, is how much of the mineral is calcium and how much is phosphorus, which builds a weaker, more brittle bone. Because the bisphosphonates discourage new bone growth, the bone becomes older and more brittle. Any new bone the body manages to lay down is constructed with more phosphorus than calcium, which produces a weaker, more brittle bone.

Phosphorus is an extremely caustic substance. If you dropped a chunk of pure phosphorus on a wooden or plastic table, the mineral would eat through the surface. The phosphorus in bisphosphonates has a similar, caustic effect in the digestive tract. Patients are told to sit upright for at least 30 minutes after taking a bisphosphonate drug. If they lie down and the pill lingers in one place in the esophagus, the phosphorus can burn a hole through the esophagus. The medication may also wreak havoc farther along in the digestive tract, in the stomach and/or the intestines.

I am not totally opposed to using bisphosphonates. They are, however, my last choice in treating osteoporosis. Some women with severe osteoporosis cannot supplement hormones, e.g., after breast, uterine or ovarian cancer. For these women, bisphosphonates may be a viable alternative.

Some women (and their physicians) think they can take a bisphosphonate and then forget about any of the preceding steps to support bone health. These medications will not excuse you from making good lifestyle choices. I've had several patients who have come to me after taking a bisphosphonate for a year *who still have significant bone loss.*

I intentionally use the term "additive" approach to bone health because some women can support bone health with diet and exercise alone. Others need to add supplements and some need all four steps. Jumping to Step 4, however, cannot replace eating well, exercising and ensuring that you have the nutrients needed to build strong bones.

HOT FLASHES

One of the most common symptoms of perimenopause and menopause is hot flashes. Eighty percent of women in this culture experience hot flashes. In other cultures, the reverse is true. The Japanese language, for example, has no word for "hot flash."

I had a patient who came to me for support with hot flashes and other menopausal symptoms. She was frustrated that her older, Asian female gynecologist seemed to have no understanding of her menopausal symptoms.

"I mean, she looked at me like I was from *Mars*," said the exasperated woman.

I smiled and shrugged my shoulders. "She probably, literally, didn't understand what you were talking about. In Asian cultures, women have few, if any, hot flashes. From her reaction, I'd say she's one of the women who never had hot flashes."

Why are women living in Asian and more traditional cultures relatively free of menopausal symptoms? Several factors play a role:

Most women living in Asia and traditional cultures eat primarily local, whole foods. Big Macs, Hamburger Helper and instant mashed potatoes are not the foundation of their diet. The more nutritious your diet and the more individualized for your particular body, the fewer hot flash symptoms you are likely to have.

Wine, other alcoholic drinks and coffee all have heating effects in the body. I'm referring to the energetic properties, NOT the literal temperature of the drink. Iced coffee, for example still has a heating effect on the body. The more internal heat, the greater the number of hot flashes

Exercise is vitally important for stress reduction, relaxing sleep and bone health. In addition, regular exercise reduces the number of hot flashes. Women who exercise three hours over the course of a week have 70-percent fewer hot flashes. Most Asian women do not have to join a gym to exercise; physical movement comes with the daily activities in their lives.

Phytoestrogens—weak, plant-based estrogens that mimic our own—can reduce hot flash symptoms. Most Asian women eat a significant amount of soy, one of the most common phytoestrogen-rich foods. Other examples of phytoestrogen-rich plants are flaxseeds, pomegranate, red clover, dong quai (*Angelica sinensis*) and black cohosh. Including some soy, flax and/or pomegranate in the diet on a daily basis can be very helpful in smoothing the hormonal transition through peri-menopause into menopause.

Vary your intake of phytoestrogens. The greater amount you eat of any one particular food and the more often, the more likely you are to develop intolerance to that food. In this culture, we have a tremendous number of soy additives in our diet—textured vegetable protein, soy lecithin, soy isolates and soy sauce. The list goes on and on. Asian women have some soy each day but *not* huge quantities.

Personal and cultural attitudes about aging have a profound effect on women's experience of menopause. Most women in this culture feel they are *losing* something during menopause. They may fear (or actually experience) the loss of their job, career, health, primary relationships and social stature. Many women report they suddenly feel invisible. "I didn't realize until menopause that I was used to being looked at in a certain way. After menopause, that all stopped. I suddenly felt like *no one* was looking at me."

In contrast, women *and* men in Asian cultures would be gaining in stature and respect at this time in their lives. In the Philippines, for example, a 60th birthday party is more noteworthy than a "sweet sixteen" party. At 60, someone is an honored elder in the community, sought out for advice and wise counsel.

Imagine living in a culture where age was welcomed, even revered! I sense that the Baby Boomers will be transforming our understanding of age, just as we have transformed every phase of the life cycle. Only when the Baby Boomers entered menopause did the words "hot flash," "vaginal dryness" and "hormone replacement therapy" become household words. The women of earlier generations either breezed through menopause or suffered in silence. Their physicians, too, were impotent in helping with the major physical, mental and emotional changes that accompanied menopause. "The Change" was not well understood and certainly not well-supported in the medical community.

I should note here that I do prescribe hormone replacement therapy but only in very specific situations. I evaluate each woman as an individual instead of making blanket decisions like, "All women should be on hormones," or "No women should take hormones." The two main reasons that have legitimate medical support are severe osteoporosis/bone loss and menopausal symptoms that are severe enough to disrupt daily functions.

For women who are taking progesterone, estrogen and/or testosterone for acute menopausal symptoms, my aim is to help them stabilize and then *wean off* the hormones. In Europe, HRT is rarely prescribed for more than six months. Menopause is considered a normal, natural life transition and the body is supported only for a short period—just long enough to ease the transition.

For bone loss, estrogen helps *maintain* bone, while testosterone and possibly progesterone stimulate osteoblasts—the cells that lay down new bone. For women with severe osteoporosis, they usually take hormone replacement therapy for the rest of their lives.

The point here is that menopause is a normal, healthy life transition. I have read some of the authors who suggest that we should continue to have repro-ductive-age hormone levels for the rest of our lives. If we *really* wanted to be youthful, why not return to the hormonal levels of a six- or seven-year-old? And, in fact, that is precisely what we do as we transition through peri-menopause into menopause. Our levels are quite similar to children's hormonal levels and steady instead of cyclic, as we were as young girls.

Hot flashes from Chinese medical perspective

As mentioned earlier, most Asian languages do not have a word for hot flash. Chinese medicine has a deep understanding, however, of night sweats and heat flushes. Remember that the Chinese think of the body being a balance of *yin* (nourishing, cooling, fluid aspects) and *yang* (warming, heating, activating properties). Think of *yin* as an iron kettle filled with water and *yang* as a fire below the kettle. When *yin* and *yang* are in balance, the fire heats the water, and gentle steam rises to nourish the organs. The "seat" or "bank account" of all *yin* and *yang* in the body is the kidneys, near the base of the abdomen.

By the time we are 40 years old, most of us have "spent" at least half of our inherited *yin*. We have also spent some of the *yang* but, in the West, we particu-larly spend *yin*. All of our doing, doing, doing and thinking, thinking, thinking "burn up" the yin. In this situation, the body heat increases *not* because the fire is hotter, but because the coolant is lower.

Think of a radiator in a car with low coolant fluid. The engine overheats not because there is more heat in the engine, but, rather, because the coolant is low. Similarly, menopausal women have hot flashes because of diminished *yin*, NOT because of a resurgence of *yang*.

Yang predominates during daylight hours, when we are working and active. *Yin* predominates at night, when we are resting and rejuvenating. If *yin* is diminished or "deficient," however, it cannot cool and nourish the body. Instead, the body heats up, particularly in the late afternoon and then through the night. As a result, night sweats are more common, initially, during meno-pause, usually followed later by hot flashes in the day as well. Conversely, as the body readjusts and completes the passage into menopause, hot flashes usually resolve before night sweats.

Yin deficiency in the heart can also lead to sleep disturbances. The Chinese describe sleep as our spirit resting in our heart, like a bird returning to its nest at night. If the heart is heated or agitated (figuratively, NOT literally), then we do not rest as well.

The Chinese treat insomnia, hot flashes and night sweats by nourishing *yin* with herbs, acupuncture, qigong and meditation.

- Exercise aerobically at least three hours total in a week. Aim for your target heart rate: [(220 – your age ____) – resting heart rate ____] x .65 + resting heart rate. Aerobic exercise will also reduce blood pressure, another common concern for many menopausal women.

- Avoid coffee, black tea and alcohol. According to Chinese dietary recommendations, these substances are "heating" in the body. Increased heat in the body generates hot flashes and night sweats and interrupts sleep.

- Eat phytoestrogen-rich foods on a daily basis, e.g., flaxseeds, soy and/or red clover tea.

- Seek herbal and/or acupuncture treatment with a Chinese medical practitioner. The treatments and herbs will address the root imbalances that contribute to your menopausal symptoms, rather than covering up the symptoms.

- If you choose hormone replacement therapy, use the friendliest forms of hormones, bio-identical hormones (those that exactly duplicate the hormones our own body makes). Transdermal (skin) or sublingual (under the tongue) dosing requires lower amounts of hormones than oral dosing for the same effect.

- Most conventional physicians prescribe estrogen for severe hot flashes. Consider first using bio-identical progesterone, a reproductive hormone that drops more precipitously than estrogen, even before menopause in some women. A study at the University of Pennsylvania medical school demonstrated that 70 percent of women using bio-identical progesterone had a reduction or cessation of hot flashes.

- *Any* change in hormone levels, up *or* down, can trigger hot flashes. In other words, when some women begin hormone replacement therapy or change another hormone dose, such as thyroid, hot flashes may worsen. Stay with the new dosage for at least two-to-four weeks before deciding if the prescription is appropriate.

- Create a celebration to honor this major life transition. Remember that your own personal attitudes about aging will have a profound impact on your experience of menopause and, therefore, your symptoms.

- Choose to surround yourself with juicy, creative, active older women, who welcome the changes you are undergoing and honor your special gifts and talents.

LOW LIBIDO

Recently the Vermont Country Store added "intimate massagers" to their regular offerings. Traditionally a catalogue that appealed to the older generation, filled with hard-to-find, vintage products, the offerings have gradually shifted as the founder's sons have taken the helm as chief proprietors. Like so many of his peers in the Boomer generation, Lyman Orton has brought aging and sex, one of our cultural taboos, out of the closet:

"By 2030, the population of Americans over the age of 65 will double! But as we get older, we don't have to become less able. Here at The Vermont Country Store, we take a practical, no-nonsense approach to keeping you healthy—physically, emotionally and . . . well . . . sexually, too!

"I initially offered these Intimate Solutions products because I had the merchant's sense that many of you would rather buy them from us than run down to Sex World or visit some uncomfortable Web site. Turns out my instincts were right.

"But—and here's the key—it's not about sex. It's about Aging Well, about fully embracing all that life offers as we age."

Women in the Boomer generation began to talk about menstruation and then hot flashes and menopause. These active, vital Boomer men and women now are approaching the fountain of age with the expectation that they will continue to be sexually active, enjoying their physical bodies well beyond youth and into their mature years.

Many factors influence our sexual interest, especially as we age. Our core vitality and physical energy are the foundation for supporting normal sexual interest. From both Chinese and naturopathic perspectives, the body invests its vitality first in the organs that are most important to sustain itself. You cannot live, for example, without the lungs or the liver. You can survive, however, without your reproductive organs. Of course, the species won't survive without the ability to reproduce, but these organs are not important for our immediate, personal survival.

When the body is undernourished or extremely stressed, the reproductive organs shut down. When I lived in rural India, most of the young Western women I knew had stopped menstruating. The extreme physical demands of living in a rural, Third World country had stressed the body enough to shut down the menstrual cycle.

Similarly, the body must be well-rested and well-nourished to support sexual activity. When patients report they have low libido and want to increase their sexual activity, I let them know we will be working to increase overall health and vitality to support libido. Some of the herbs that increase circulation in the lower pelvic area can help increase sexual sensations and increase enjoyment. They cannot, however, substitute for the vital energy needed to sustain healthy libido.

Libido and emotional connection

Emotional connection with our partner also contributes greatly to sexual desire. Unresolved emotional conflict—within themselves or with their partner—is one of the biggest dampers on sexual activity, especially for women.

Sadly, millions of adults in this country have experienced sexual abuse. The U.S. Department of Health and Human Services Administration for Children and Families receives approximately 2 million confirmed cases of child abuse annually, and 9.1 percent of these children are victims of sexual abuse. That means state Child Protective Services *discover and report* approximately 182,000 children who are sexually abused each year. The actual numbers likely are much higher.

Many people respond to sexual abuse by shutting down their own sexuality. Sex has become associated with power and control, not love and connection. Some women and men initially "work out" their past history of abuse through promiscuity. Later, when involved in a safe, supportive partnership, the past history of abuse may surface and the pattern may flip to the opposite extreme and an individual may have *no* interest in sex.

With patience and support, people can move through their past history and re-establish connection with their own body. Many women with a past history of sexual abuse say they don't have much physical sensation during intercourse. Most have learned to physically and emotionally disconnect from their bodies during sexual activity. Profound healing comes from learning to be in the body and experience both connection and pleasure with their partner.

Women who have never been sexually abused may also suffer with this lack of sensation and pleasure during intercourse. Some of the exercises below can help you to establish a sense of union with your own body, as well as with your partner.

How much is enough?

Cultural expectations also influence our sexuality. When I was completing my internship in the clinic, I followed the case of a woman in her early twenties who had come for treatment of low libido. She faithfully implemented the treatment suggestions offered but, after a couple of visits, she reported no change in her sexual desire.

Finally, the intern working with her asked how often she was having sex. "Oh, once a day," she reported.

"And that's not enough for your boyfriend?" asked the intern.

"Oh, no. He's in a rock 'n roll band and has a really high sex drive. He wants to have sex at least three times a day. I'm just not that interested and that's creating a lot of conflict in our relationship."

Part of this young woman's treatment involved educating her about what is "normal" for most people. In Chinese medicine, having intercourse two or three times a *week*, not per day, is considered normal.

Of course, everyone has different levels of overall vitality and, thus, sexual desire. Sexual activity also tends to change as a romantic relationship progresses. From Chinese medical perspective, too much sex drains *jing*, our inherited vitality. This inherited energy is stored in the kidneys, which in turn gives support to the lower back and knees. If the kidneys' "bank account" of energy is drained, we tend to have more low back and knee pain, as well as decreased overall vitality.

When someone is suffering with a chronic illness, the Chinese doctor usually recommends curtailing sexual activity, especially during the recovery phase. Many of the qigong students practicing with Professor Chen in Portland, Oregon were cancer patients. One woman was making a strong comeback after several rounds of chemotherapy and radiation for breast cancer. Her qigong practice was helping to rebuild her vitality and restore body systems that had been damaged by her cancer treatments. After about nine months, though, she began to worsen again.

Professor Chen took her aside to ask what had changed in her life.

The woman looked sheepish. "I know you told me not to have sex while I was rebuilding my energy, but my husband just couldn't wait any longer. He has needs, too. So we started having sex again."

Chen scheduled a private talk with this woman and her husband.

"You love your wife, don't you?" she asked the husband.

He nodded.

"And you understand that having sex weakens her vitality?"

He nodded again.

"You want your wife to live, to recover from the cancer. So, please, don't have sex with her until she has fully recovered. Can you do that?"

The husband agreed to support his wife by curtailing sex until she was clear of the cancer. Of course, stopping sex does *not* mean avoiding cuddling and other forms of intimacy. Physical contact deeply nurtures both partners, whether that intimacy leads to intercourse or not.

Treatment suggestions for low libido

- Begin making love several days before you have intercourse. This "lovemaking" might include leaving romantic phone messages for your partner, buying flowers, cuddling or writing a poem.

- Schedule dates that include time for sex. Before having children, this sort of planned lovemaking seemed cold-hearted and unromantic to me. Now, juggling work and children, I appreciate these scheduled times when I know I can relax and fully enjoy being with my partner.

- Increase daily physical intimacy. This ongoing, loving contact builds the foundation for a healthy, vital sexual connection.

- Devote plenty of time to foreplay, especially as you age and/or your relationship matures. Women take longer for vaginal tissue to lubricate and prepare for intercourse than men require for an erection. Most women's sexual response is even slower after menopause. Devote plenty of time to foreplay and stimulation before intercourse (usually a minimum of 10 to 30 minutes).

- Sexual interest usually is high for the first 24to-36 months of a relationship. According to Dr. Patricia Love, Ed.D., author of *Hot Monogamy* (Reed Business Information, Inc., 1994), certain hormones surge when we first fall in love. The body dumps these feel-good hormones into the bloodstream every time we think of our beloved *or* are in his or her presence. We think about our partner constantly, call her frequently and touch him at every opportunity. All of this mental and physical contact ensures high levels of these euphoria-producing hormones, especially during the first six months of a relationship. After six months, these hormones begin to diminish, until finally, 24-to-36 months after the beginning of the relationship, hormones return to their usual levels.

Dr. Love points out that this 36-month period is the international average for most marriages. Biologically, the timing makes sense: Three years is just long enough to fall in love, get pregnant, have a child and raise the child to toddler stage. From this point forward, mother and child are capable of survival on their own.

Dr. Love's book, *Hot Monogamy*, encourages couples to nurture their sexual interest and vitality after this three-year period. In essence, you can ride the hormonal "wave" at the beginning of a relationship. After three years, a couple usually needs to focus more on romance and friendship to fuel the sexual spark. For long-term relationships, the fire of ongoing sexual interest and vitality requires careful tending and frequent feeding.

MENSTRUAL CRAMPING

From Chinese medical perspective, stagnation leads to pain. Stagnation may be caused by cold or, paradoxically, by a decrease in the cooling, nourishing *yin* fluids of the body. A deficiency of blood, a *yin* substance, causes irritation, cramping and scanty blood flow. The deficiency is a qualitative decrease in blood, not a quantitative deficiency that would show up on a blood test.

Generally, cramping worsens with cold, whether the source of the cold is internal or external. Hong Jin, one of my professors in acupuncture school, was a renowned gynecologist in China and now lectures to gynecologists in the United States. In one of her presentations, Jin mentioned that patients who drink ice water the week before their period is due often have much more severe menstrual cramps. One of the gynecologists in the audience, a friend of Professor Jin's, scoffed at the idea of ice water causing cramping. The week before *her* period, she left a pitcher of water in the refrigerator and drank nothing but ice water.

When her bleeding began, the gynecologist humbly called Professor Jin to report that she had the worst menstrual cramps of her life.

From Western medical perspective, menstrual cramping usually is associated with estrogen dominance, or too much estrogen and not enough progesterone activity. Progesterone has a relaxing effect on smooth muscle, including the uterus. Endometriosis, the migration of the endometrial lining to other areas of the body, can also cause menstrual cramping. Usually, the endometrial tissue migrates to the lower abdominal region. Rarely, the tissue is found in other areas.

I have worked with women who have bleeding from their nose and one in her lungs, with every menstrual cycle. The current medical theory suggests the tissue "migrates" when we are adults. I suspect the tissue did not migrate correctly much earlier, during embryonic development. Hormonal changes as we enter our adult years trigger these misplaced tissues to grow and "shed," causing bleeding in unexpected places.

- Supplement bio-identical progesterone from ovulation to menses (usually the last 14 days of the menstrual cycle). This is the time the ovaries normally make progesterone, so you are simply augmenting the body's normal production. Choosing transdermal (skin) applications of hormones reduces the amount of hormone you need. The average oral dose of bio-identical progesterone, for example, is 200 mg daily. An equivalent transdermal dose is 40 mg daily. I highly recommend Emerita Pro-Gest, the only bio-identical progesterone cream that has had pharmacological absorption testing and other double-blind, placebo controlled tests.

  - For reproductive-age women, use ¼ teaspoon of Emerita Pro-Gest twice a day, *from ovulation to menses.* STOP when your menstrual bleeding begins. Rub into the smooth, hairless areas (abdomen, chest, inner arms) and rotate application site daily.
  - For peri-menopausal women (who are not necessarily ovulating every cycle), use ¼ teaspoon Emerita Pro-Gest twice a day, *all the days you are not bleeding.* STOP when your menstrual bleeding begins. Rub into the smooth, hairless areas (abdomen, chest, inner arms) and rotate application site daily.

- Avoid cold foods and drinks the week before menses begins. Cold causes constriction and exacerbates cramping, whether the source of the cold is internal (food and drink) or external (cold drafts, swimming in cold water, etc.).
- Exercise is a good preventive, increasing circulation and decreasing stagnation.
- Clear your schedule as much as possible the day before you begin bleeding. If possible, have a completely quiet, unscheduled day when you begin bleeding.

Botanical therapy:
- Yarrow (*Achillea millefolium*) – acts as a diuretic for bloating associated with premenstrual syndrome (PMS).
- Wild yam (*Discorea villosa*) – reduces cramping (smooth muscle relaxant). Wild yam also has phytoestrogen effect, which can help to *lower* overall estrogen activity in reproductive-age women. Wild yam will *not* convert to progesterone in the body; this conversion must take place in a laboratory.

- Valerian (*Valeriana officinalis*) – to reduce cramping and relax smooth muscles. (The uterus is smooth muscle tissue.)
- Red raspberry leaf (*Rubus idaeus*) – uterine tonic.

Combine equal parts of the above. Drink three-to-four cups of tea per day, or take two dropperfuls every one-to-two hours during acute, severe cramping.

- False Unicorn Root (*Chamaelirium luteum/Helonius dioica*) —increases leutenizing hormone (LH) secretion in the pituitary, which in turn increases progesterone production.
  - Dose: 30-to-60 drops, 1-to-4 times a day.

Nutritional therapy:

- Increase fiber in the diet. Slow, sluggish bowels encourage the re-uptake of hormones the body is trying to excrete through the intestines. High hormonal levels may exacerbate menstrual cramping, as well as PMS symptoms.
- Drink at least two quarts of water per day to increase elimination from the body.
- Eat magnesium-rich foods. Magnesium encourages muscle relaxation.
- Take 50-to-100 mg of vitamin B6 per day for at least two months.
- Exercise aerobically at least 20 minutes, four times per week. Exercise increases circulation in the reproductive organs and decreases stress levels, both of which can decrease menstrual cramping.

Homeopathic remedies: 30c potency

- Belladonna – heavy sensation in abdomen. Menses bright red, profuse. Restless. Head sensitive to drafts. Feels worse after jarring or even when touched.
- Borax – fears downward motion. Membrane and tissue pass with menses. Early, profuse bleeding, with colic and nausea. Application of pressure eases discomfort. Feels better during cold weather.
- Bryonia – "vicarious menses," i.e., nosebleed rather than menstrual flow. Inter-menses pains with pelvic and abdominal soreness. Avoids the least motion. Thirsty for large amounts of water.
- Calcarea phosphorica – violent backache. Chilly. Menses is early, excessive, bright red; occurs every two weeks.

- Chamomilla – dark, clotted blood with labor-like pains. Irritable, cross, quarrelsome. Thirsty. Feels worse at night, when angry, or after drinking coffee.
- Colocynthis – Pain better bending over double; pain "bores into" ovary. Pain eases with pressure. Restless. Waves of violent, gripping pain.
- Magnesium phosphoricum (Mag phos) – cramps that are relieved with warmth, e.g., a hot water bottle over the abdomen.
- Pulsatilla – sensation of band around throat just before menses. Clotted, intermittent, changeable menses.

When to consult a physician

- If severe menstrual cramping occurs more than twice in a year
- If menstrual cramping worsens over time (possible indication that endometriosis may be developing)
- If the cramps are severe enough to stop your daily activities

NAUSEA IN PREGNANCY

Often one of the earliest signals that you are pregnant is gnawing, low-grade nausea. Of course, this symptom is *not* a requirement during pregnancy. Some women breeze through their entire pregnancy with no nausea whatsoever. Other women are nauseated for nine months. Your experience during each pregnancy will be unique. During one pregnancy, for example, you may have no nausea while, during another, you may have nausea during the first trimester.

Nausea and eating

Working with nausea during pregnancy is counter-intuitive, because the best way to reduce or avoid nausea is to eat. This is just the opposite of what you normally would do if you were feeling queasy.

Blood sugar fluctuations are the primary cause of nausea during pregnancy. Perhaps our bodies are so exquisitely sensitive to blood sugar drops because these lapses in blood sugar can potentially hamper the fetus' development. The steadier your blood sugar, the less difficulty you will have with nausea during pregnancy.

Of course, you may have such severe nausea you simply cannot eat, or you may be able to eat only at certain times of the day. Take advantage of your "clear" periods to eat as well and as much as you can.

Carrying twins, for example, I was usually nauseated until about 4 p.m. I ate as much healthy food as I could during the evening. I snacked during the morning and early afternoon, when the nausea was at its worst.

Eat the healthiest foods possible. The only food a colleague's wife could keep down during her first trimester was chocolate ice cream. She chose the highest quality, organic ice cream she could find. Knowing the importance of optimal nutrition during pregnancy, she discussed the situation with her physician.

Her obstetrician smiled. "Your baby will be just fine. Just keep eating what you can."

Thankfully, this woman did deliver a gorgeous, perfectly healthy little girl. In fact, her daughter smelled of roses for the first month of her life. In the Hindu and Catholic traditions, many saints smell of roses. They simply exude the scent from their bodies. Who knows? Perhaps chocolate ice cream added to this baby's saintly attributes.

Of course, eating ice cream alone is not an ideal solution to nausea during pregnancy. I offer this story to illustrate how resourceful our bodies are in nourishing the developing fetus. *Your body will choose in favor of nourishing the fetus*, up to the point of literal starvation. Your dietary choices are meant to support the fetus, as well as minimize damage to your own body. Your body, for example, will pull calcium from your bones to support the baby's development if you are not eating enough calcium in your diet.

Treatment suggestions

- Practice "preventative eating," meaning that you eat regularly, when you are not nauseated. The nausea usually will improve eating easy to digest foods, such as crackers or warm soup.
- Eat protein every two hours. You don't need to eat a 12-ounce steak every two hours. A handful of nuts and an apple, or a small bowl of bean soup, will suffice.
- Avoid very sweet, fatty, greasy or rich foods. Cold foods paralyze the digestive tract. The stomach has to warm up before it can resume digesting the food. From Chinese medical perspective, these "damp-forming" foods will worsen the symptoms. This makes sense from Western medical perspective as well, because fatty, rich foods tax the liver and gallbladder, also contributing to digestive upsets. The story above, of the woman who ate nothing but chocolate ice cream for the entire first trimester, completely contradicts this information. That's

the mystery of pregnancy! Most women have *more* nausea, not less, after eating fatty, rich and/or cold foods.

- Eat simple, highly nutritious foods. Breakfast, for example, might be wholegrain crackers and a few nuts. A couple of hours later eat a small bowl of bean soup. Steamed vegetables, whole grain rice and fish or beans make a great lunch. Give the stomach small, regular "doses" of food.

- Prepare a box or basket of food that you can carry with you during the day. Ideally, these foods would keep and travel well and contain significant amounts of protein to help stabilize your blood sugar. Eating sugary, processed foods will simply cause a spike and drop in your blood sugar levels, thereby aggravating your nausea. Take the box to work, or leave it in the back seat of the car if you are driving or running errands. Some foods to consider, that travel well:

  - whole grain crackers
  - instant hummus
  - Taste Adventure™ instant soups
  - canned sardines
  - canned tuna
  - fresh, unsalted nuts
  - nut butter (almond, hazelnut, sunflower butter. If possible, avoid peanut butter, the most difficult of the nut butters to digest)
  - apples (eat some nuts with the apple)

- Herbs for nausea: Drink these herbs as tea, or dilute alcohol tinctures of the herbs in water. Diluted in water, the small amount of alcohol will not hurt the baby. If you are traveling or working, the tinctures are easier to carry with you and prepare.

  - Chamomile (*Matricaria rescutita*) reduces spasms and inflammation and calms the stomach. Chamomile will ease nausea, gas and stomach pain. This gentle but very effective herb is even safe for babies who are having trouble relaxing and falling asleep. Chamomile also has some calming and sedating effect on the nervous system. Drinking chamomile may make you sleepy, so drink sparingly early in the day. *Caution: Avoid chamomile if you have known allergies to plants in the Asteraceae family (formerly called the Compositae family).*

  - Ginger (*Zingiber officinalis*) warms and soothes the stomach and reduces burping and flatulence. You can safely drink two or three cups of ginger tea per day. If you do not respond well to ginger tea, try using ginger tincture. Take 20-30 drops three times a day, with food. You can dilute the tincture in a cup of warm or room temperature water. *Caution: Large doses are contraindicated in pregnancy*, based on the potential to depress the central nervous system and cause heart arrhythmias. This research was conducted on animals, not humans.

- AVOID peppermint (*Mentha piperita*), which relaxes the lower esophageal sphincter, thereby encouraging acid reflux. Peppermint is also an emmenagogue, meaning that it encourages the shedding of the uterine lining, which definitely is contraindicated during pregnancy. You may use peppermint during pregnancy under the guidance of a qualified health care provider, i.e., one trained in medical herbalism.

- Wear a bracelet that stimulates Pericardium 6, an acupuncture point known to calm the stomach. These bracelets are sold for motion sickness as well as nausea in pregnancy. Sea Band™ makes these in adult and children's sizes.
- Acupuncture can help reduce nausea and other early pregnancy symptoms.
- Studies have demonstrated that regular acupuncture during the pregnancy can help ease labor and delivery. I recently worked with a patient who had acupuncture at least once a month during her pregnancy. She had delivered three other children, but she had to be induced with Pitocin for all three of those deliveries. With acupuncture and other supportive therapies, she was able to dilate and deliver her fourth baby with no interventions. She came to the clinic the afternoon before she delivered in labor, hoping that the acupuncture would stimulate her body to have stronger contractions. In the past, she would begin labor and then the contractions would "fizzle out." She was 5 cm dilated when she arrived at the clinic. After the treatment, the contractions seemed to stop. When she went into the hospital four hours later, however, she was 9 cm dilated, almost ready to push. In that four hour period, she had painlessly dilated from 5 to 9 cm!
- In addition to Pericardium 6, you can use acupressure on the following point to reduce nausea: Stomach 36 (see Acupressure in Chapter 2 for point location).

- Homeopathic remedies can ease nausea during pregnancy without harming the fetus in any way. Remember that you may need a different remedy at different times if your symptoms change:

  - Nux vomica: nausea in the morning and after eating. Heartburn, nausea and vomiting. The stomach is sensitive to pressure, e.g., leaning against a counter. Violent vomiting. Chilly. Worse pressure of clothes, in the morning, in cold air, coffee. Better in the evening, resting, napping.

  - Sepia: Severe nausea, especially in the morning. "All gone" feeling that does not improve with eating. Craves vinegar and pickles. Indifferent about other family members and their needs. Worse in the morning, cold air, sexual excesses, before a thunderstorm. Better from strenuous exercise, cold drinks, pressure, sleep.

  - Tabacum: incessant nausea; worse from tobacco smoke. Vomiting during pregnancy, with lots of spitting. Terrible, faint feeling in the pit of the stomach. Very despondent, discontented, forgetful. Worse in the evening, worse moving. Better with cold, fresh air, uncovering the abdomen, at twilight.

  - Kreosotum: vomits food several hours after eating. Cold feeling in the stomach. Vomit is very acidic and excoriates the mouth. Worse lying down, cold, at night (6 p.m.-to-6 a.m.) Better with warmth, movement, hot food.

  - Phosphorus: craves cold food and drinks, but vomits as soon as the cold drink warms in the stomach. Vomits food soon after swallowing. Worse lying on the left side or back. Worse from emotional upsets, warm food, salty foods, weather changes. Better lying on the right side OR sitting up. Better after eating, sleep and massage.

PROSTATITIS

Prostatitis means inflammation ("-*itis*") of the prostate gland. This condition is one of the most common concerns male patients in my practice report. About 30 percent of men have difficulty with urination by age 50. Before this age, most urination problems are the result of infections. Sometimes acute prostate infections can lead to chronic urinary symptoms, such as burning with urination, increased frequency of urination and low-grade irritating pain in the perineal area.

Occasionally, men have low-grade infections for years, with no symptoms to alert them to the infection. Caused by a variety of bacteria, prostate infections are more common in men who have had more sexual activity, especially with multiple sexual partners.

When the prostate is enlarged, you may feel like you are sitting on a ball and have to shift your position frequently when sitting. You may have difficulty starting a stream of urine, or the urine may flow more slowly. Lower abdominal pressure or pain is common, as is more frequent urination at night. If the inflammation is very severe, you may have pain with urination and even a fever. Be sure to see your family doctor for a urinalysis to eliminate the possibility of a bladder infection, which can cause similar symptoms (pain with urination, frequent urination, lower abdominal pain and fever). If you have a urinary tract infection, the infection must be treated before you begin any prostate treatments. If the urinalysis shows no infection, then you can move forward with suggestions for treating prostate inflammation.

Prostatitis and xenoestrogen exposure

Like breast and ovarian cancer, prostate cancer rates are skyrocketing in the U.S. This trend is not surprising, considering the increasing load of toxic chemicals in the environment. All petroleum-based chemicals act like estrogen in the body. "*Xeno*" means "foreign," so xenoestrogens are chemicals that act like estrogen in the body. Estrogen's message for reproductive tissues (prostate, testicles, breasts, ovaries, uterus) is "divide, divide, divide; don't bother maturing, just keep dividing." At the very least, these chemicals cause overgrowth of tissues, leading to an enlarged prostate gland. Cancer cells are extremely rapidly dividing cells. If estrogen's "grow, grow, grow" message continues long enough, the cells edge in the direction of cancer.

Just in the last week I had a new patient in his early thirties who already had signs of prostate enlargement. His visit was to treat chronic pain from a work-related injury. I always ask about overall health, even with musculoskeletal injuries. From both Chinese and naturopathic perspectives, all of the body systems need to be working well in order to support tissue repair. I was surprised to see on his intake chart that at 33 years of age he already had urinary problems.

When I asked whether he had had a prostate exam, he replied, "Yeah, they did an exam and found a nodule on my prostate. But, after the testing, they said it was nothing to worry about. They would just watch it."

"Have you had any significant chemical exposures?" I asked. "Like petroleum products, or agricultural fertilizers and insecticides?"

He smiled and nodded. "Yeah, *lots.*"

We talked about the effect of these chemicals in the body and how they increase estrogen activity. Twenty years ago the conventional thinking about prostate enlargement was that increased testosterone levels stimulate prostate overgrowth. The current, deeper understanding of hormones also points toward estrogen for stimulating prostate overgrowth. Both estrogen and testosterone are "anabolic" steroid hormones, meaning they stimulate cell growth. As men age, testosterone levels drop while estrogen levels remain steady *or* increase. Estrogen, in essence, is "unmasked." (Women have the opposite scenario as they age: Testosterone levels stay steady or increase while estrogen and progesterone drop).

When the body is exposed to petrochemicals, fertilizers, off-gassing from plastics, etc., the liver clears what it can at the time. What the body is unable to metabolize and excrete is stored in fat and lymphatic tissue.

Each body can tolerate a certain amount of chemical exposure. I use the metaphor of a trash can: each of us has a different sized trash can, representing the amount of chemical exposure we can tolerate. What you cannot immediately clear ends up in the trash can—in this case, fat and lymph storage in the body. Most of us have repeated, small exposures of chemicals.

Occasionally, I work with patients who have one massive chemical exposure that immediately fills that "trash can," or tolerable backlog of chemical exposure. For most, though, the trash can fills slowly, imperceptibly, over time. Suddenly, though, when the trash can is full, you begin to experience the symptoms of xenoestrogen exposure. I say "suddenly" because the body has been able to tolerate the slowly accumulating backlog of waste up until that time. Think of that final, small exposure like the straw that broke the camel's back.

The constellation of physical conditions associated with excess exposure to solvents, petrochemicals, chloro- and fluorocarbons is called "environmental illness." In this case, we are talking about a specific side effect of chemical exposure: overgrowth of the prostate gland and possibly prostate cancer.

Obviously other factors can contribute to prostatitis as well.

Those include:

- Venereal diseases, such as gonorrhea, syphilis and Chlamydia infection. Just as the bladder can become infected with a bacterial overgrowth, the prostate can as well.
- Coffee: known to irritate the bladder lining, coffee can also affect the prostate.

How to support prostate health

First and foremost, eliminate as many chemical exposures as possible.

- Wear gloves when working with petrochemicals, e.g., changing the oil or filling the lawnmower with gas.
- Instead of using a gas-powered lawnmower, consider finding an electric lawnmower. In 2001 a study in Sweden concluded: "Air pollution from cutting grass for an hour with a gasoline powered lawn mower is about the same as that from a 100-mile automobile ride." In other words, one hour walking behind a gasoline-driven lawnmower delivers as much toxic pollution as sitting for an hour in rush hour traffic in L.A. You absorb even more of the toxins breathing deeply as you walk behind the mower.
- Maintain an organic garden and lawn. The chemicals sprayed on lawns and gardens are extremely toxic. Control weeds by burning or spraying with 11% acetic acid vinegar (available in garden supply stores).
- Eliminate coffee.
- Eliminate simple carbohydrates—the "white wonders" such as white flour, white sugar and white rice.
- Eliminate alcohol. From Chinese medical perspective, prostatitis is caused primarily by an accumulation of "dampness" and "heat" in the "lower burner," or lower abdomen. Alcohol increases dampness and heat in the body, thereby aggravating any already established accumulation of damp and heat in the lower part of the body, i.e., the prostate.
- Eat phytoestrogen-rich foods such as seaweed, flaxseed and soy. These weak, plant-based estrogens compete with the body's stronger, internally produced estrogens for receptor sites. If you "sit" one of these weaker phytoestrogens in an estrogen receptor site, you temporarily block one of the stronger endogenous estrogens from binding at that receptor site. Phytoestrogens can help *lower* overall estrogen activity.

Botanicals for prostatitis and epididymitis

- A combination of the following three herbs helps to regulate estrogen and testosterone activity:
  - Saw palmetto (*Sabal serrulata*) contains fatty acids, vitamin E and several plant sterols that reduce inflammation. Saw palmetto slows the conversion of testosterone to its active form (dihydrotestosterone, or DHT) and inhibits the biding of 25-dihydrotestosterone to receptor sites in the prostate, thereby reducing the rate of cell division. Slowing prostate cell division reduces overgrowth (benign prostatic hypertrophy, or BPH)

and possibly prostate cancer. Remember that a cancer cell is an extremely rapidly dividing, extremely poorly developed cell, so slowing cell division protects against cancer formation. Dose: 60 drops of tincture, 2 times a day OR 3 capsules of dried herb twice a day.

- False unicorn root (*Chamaelirium luteum*): 60 drops of tincture twice daily, for at least two weeks
- Pasque flower OR wind flower (*Anemone pulsatilla*): 30 drops of tincture three times a day for men with epididymitis. Combine with parsley and goldenseal for treating prostatitis.
- For prostate infection
  - Partridgeberry (*Mitchella repens*): for painful and/or decreased urine flow, partridgeberry will also address prostatitis. Combine with goldenseal (*Hydrastis*) for urethritis (inflammation of the urethra)
- Another treatment for prostatitis is a combination of
  - Pasque flower (*Anemone pulsatilla*)
  - Goldenseal (*Hydrastis canadensis*)
  - Parsley (*Petroselinium sativum*)
  - Combine *equal* parts of these three tinctures and take 90 drops three times a day.

Nutrients

- Zinc: This nutrient improves immune function and normalizes reductase enzyme function in the prostate. For the first month, take 100 mg per day; then, reduce the dose to 50 mg per day as a maintenance dose.
- Essential fatty acids help to run the anti-inflammatory pathways in the body, particularly the omega-3 essential fatty acids. The richest sources of omega-3 fatty acids are flaxseed oil and hemp oil. Take 1 tablespoon per day for a week; then reduce to 1 teaspoon per day as a maintenance dose.

NOTE: Always take any supplemental oils with protein, which polarizes the fat molecules so that they can be absorbed across the intestines. If you take any kind of oil on an empty stomach OR with a meal with little protein (e.g. a salad), the oil will pass through the intestines without being absorbed.

Essential oils

Combine the following essential oils in 2 tablespoons of vegetable oil (olive, sesame, apricot, etc.) Massage the oil into the lower abdomen and lower back twice a day, to reduce inflammation in the prostate gland. Several of these essential oils have anti-microbial properties as well.

- lavender (*Lavendula officinalis*), 5 drops
- cypress (*Cupressus sempervirens*), 10 drops
- *Eucalyptus radiata,* 10 drops (make sure you are using *Eucalyptus radiata*, which is milder in its effects than more commonly used *Eucalyptus globulus*)
- Thyme (*Thymus vulgarus*), 5 drops

Homeopathic remedies

- Apis: enlarged, inflamed prostate gland. Painful urination; last drop burns; colored urine; sharp, stinging pain; no thirst. Worse with heat in the room or bed; worse touch. Better cool air, motion.
- Aurum: for testicle and/or epididymus pain, particularly on the right side.
- Baryta carb: Enlarged prostate, especially in elderly; impotence; decreased sexual desire; urethral burning; hemorrhoids protrude during urination. Slow moving, very chilly. Better warm wraps, walking in the open air.
- Calcarea carbonica: enlarged prostate with frequent emissions during urination, after urination, after stool. Increased sexual desire; premature ejaculation; feels weak after intercourse. Thirsty, chilly. Worse cold, bathing, exertion. Better dry weather, lying on painful side.
- Conium: hard, enlarged prostate. Prostate fluid emission with stool, with emotions. Heavy sensation; effects of suppressed sexual appetite; stony hardness of prostate. Acute, cutting pains in the neck of the bladder. Worse celibacy, alcohol. Better letting penis hang down; better with motion and pressure.
- Lycopodium: prostate fluid emission with erection; enlarged prostate; impotence; premature ejaculation. Urine is slow to come; much flatulence; chilly. Worse pressure of clothes, particularly around the waist; 4-to-8 p.m. Better warm drinks, food, cold applications, urinating.
- Pulsatilla: enlarged prostate. Inflammation, especially from suppressed gonorrhea. Acute prostatitis, with pain and bladder spasming with urination. Thick, yellow-green discharge. Shifting symptoms. Thirstless, desires fresh air. Worse warm room, rich fatty foods, evening. Better cold, fresh, open air; gentle motion.

CHAPTER 7

Create your own roadmap to health

I cannot give you a definition of perfect health, but I can guide you in creating your own. The focus here is discovering what is important to *you*, so that you can organize your life around what matters most to you.

One of my patients defines "health" as competing in three iron-man competitions each year. Another wants enough energy to complete her work by day, paint in her studio in the evenings and ride bikes with her grandchildren.

Once you have this template for health, you can work effectively with any health care provider. She does not necessarily need to know your vision of health. You will be passing her recommendations through the "screen" of your definition of health and deciding whether or not the protocol makes sense in fulfilling your own vision of health.

Dale's story

One of my patients in the High Level Wellness Program©, for example, had decided he never wanted any heroic medical interventions to save his life. A forester by profession and a pied piper among children, Dale had a passion for teaching others about sustainable living and celebrating life on this Earth.

When Dale entered the High Level Wellness Program, he assumed the four-month program would be a "cake walk," simply affirming his already established diet and exercise program. During the initial physical exam, however, I discovered a leaky valve in his heart. After a couple of weeks of testing, the cardiologist and surgeon were not certain that Dale would survive a major surgery.

At 48-years-old, faced with the possibility of dying within a few months without surgery, Dale began to reconsider his options. His vision of health included stewarding the land where he lived and sharing his passion for the Earth with children. He recognized that, without surgery to correct the leaky heart valve, he would be unable to fulfill his dreams.

After much soul-searching, Dale decided to pursue open-heart surgery to correct the leaky valve. He chose to have the surgery in order to fulfill his commitment to the Earth. He hated the prospect of taking Coumadin—an anti-coagulant drug that compensates for the turbulent blood flow caused by the artificial heart valve—for the rest of his life.

"Taking that pill every day," he reported to the Wellness Program support group, "will remind me of my commitment to the Earth."

Thankfully, Dale survived the surgery and recovered very quickly. Now, 16 years later, he continues to work with children, introducing them to wilderness living and forestry principles.

Having created his own definition of health, Dale was equipped to make difficult life decisions when faced with a medical crisis. Without that template for health, he would have had a much more difficult time navigating the medical system.

With that definition of health, Dale assembled a team of physicians who worked together to achieve his vision of health. The cardiologist, surgeon and I developed a respectful, collaborative relationship that placed Dale and his vision of health at the center of our efforts.

What's your definition of health?

Health is more than the absence of symptoms; it is the presence of what you value most in your life.

Ask yourself: "If I had all the energy in the world and felt really great, what would I be doing? What would I be focused on? What would be important to me?" *That* is your definition of health.

Often, when I ask patients what health looks like for them, they list all of the things they think they need to do in order to be healthy. "Oh, I'd be at the gym four times a week, and I'd be eating more vegetables and cutting out sugar . . ."

"Do you really love the gym?" I ask. "Or do you think you need to go to the gym to be healthy?"

Some want to go to the gym because they love working out. For them, we place "Go to the gym four times a week" in their vision of health. For others, going to the gym is a necessary evil to feel good, maintain weight, increase muscle strength, etc.

For those who dislike the gym, I ask, "And what would you get from going to the gym?"

"Hmm, I guess I would feel more energetic. I like having the muscle tone, even though I don't like working out. And I like the sociability—you know, meeting friends at the gym after work."

"OK, so what you want is increased energy, muscle tone and time with your friends. Is that right?"

"Yes," she says, eyes brightening. "That's right."

"So, let's put those things in your vision of health. The gym may or may not be the ideal way of fulfilling those aspects of your vision. For now, we'll consider 'go to the gym four times a week' an action step that serves your vision of having energy, muscle tone and time with your friends."

Creating a road map to achieve your vision of health

In order to create the level of health you want, you need to know what health looks like *for you*. As Phyllis, my 96-year-old friend, says, "You have to know where you are going before you can buy a ticket. You can't just go to the bus station and say, 'Give me a ticket.' You have to know where you're going first. That's the ticket!"

Robert Fritz, a long-time mentor, has written several insightful books about the creative process, including *The Path of Least Resistance* (Fawcett Books, 1989) and *Creating* (Ballantine Books, 1993). Fritz developed the following paradigm for creating *anything* you want in your life. You could also use this same structure to make dinner, sew a dress, or design a business. The scale and focus is up to you. For right now, we'll focus on creating your vision of optimal health.

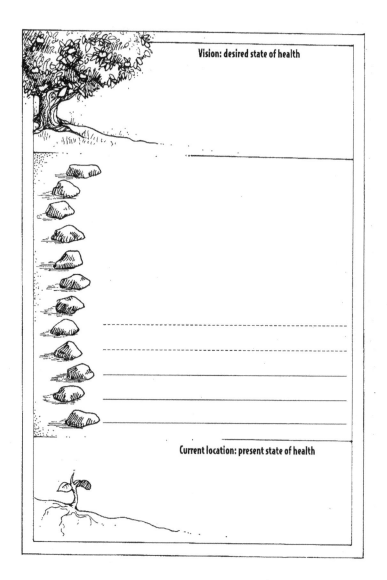

In the following exercise, complete the Journey to Health chart in seven steps:

1   Describe your destination (the state of health you desire).

2   Accurately describe your current location (your current state of health).

3   Notice the difference between where you are and where you want to be.

4   Simultaneously hold an image of your desired state and your current state of health. Notice the structural tension generated by the disparity between the two pictures.

5   Ask yourself, "If I could have my desired state of health, would I take it ?"

6   If the answer is "Yes," then CHOOSE that state of health. "I choose. . ." and describe what you desire.

7   Fill in action steps that will move you toward your destination.

1. Are you interested in being healthy?

Patients often look puzzled when I ask this question. "Of course I want to be healthy," most patients say. "Why else would I be here?"

Over the years, though, I've learned that not everyone wants to be healthy. Many want the absence of symptoms, which is different from having full, vibrant health.

When the symptoms "go away," what do you have left? Imagine a stone in the center of your palm. If that stone "went away," what would you have left? You would have the *absence* of something. In other words, you would have NOTHING.

Think of a painter approaching a canvas. She doesn't say, "How do I get rid of the problem of this empty canvas?" Instead, she focuses on the colors, shapes and forms she wants to see on the canvas.

Creating health involves bringing something into being, like the painter brushing color on the canvas. Simply eliminating something, i.e., "solving a problem" or "resolving a symptom," will not create the level of health you desire.

Of course, problem-solving can serve the artist in the creative process. The painter may need to discover a new way of applying paint, or mixing colors, to achieve a certain hue. Problem-solving alone, however, will not create anything new.

2. Define your personal vision of health.

If you do want to be healthy, what does that look like *for you*? Ask yourself: "If I had all the energy I wanted, if I felt great, what would I be doing? What would be important to me?"

Make sure you are describing the end result, not what you think you need to do to get there. Some patients, for example, begin to tell me action steps they believe they need to take in order to be healthy. "Oh, I'd be in yoga class five days a week and drinking two quarts of water a day . . ."

"Do you *love* yoga class?" I'll ask. "Or do you think you need yoga in order to be healthy?"

If someone answers she loves going to yoga class, I encourage her to add that to her vision of health. If he says, "I hate yoga; I just go to lose weight," then I encourage him to move "go to yoga class five times a week" to the "secondary choices" section in the structural tension chart. We will discuss secondary choices in more detail below.

Be sure to tell yourself the truth about what you really want.

Perhaps, at age 75, you want to dance with the New York City Ballet and you've never had a ballet lesson in your life. If you truly want to be a ballet dancer, include that in your vision of health. Although you may not wow an audience in New York, you may have a fantastic time taking ballet lessons with a local dance instructor. Taking ballet lessons is an example of a secondary choice, an important step we'll revisit below.

Trying to dilute your vision to make it "more realistic" destroys the potency of your vision. You don't know whether or not you will be able to create part or all of your vision. Telling yourself the truth about what you want relieves you of the burden of lying to yourself or trying to talk yourself out of what matters most to you.

3. Add standards of measurement.

Many people leave out important details when they envision something. When I lived in Portland, Oregon, the architect who designed the beautiful glass spires of the convention center never considered how the glass would be cleaned! He left no openings in the glass structure for maintenance.

In painting your picture of health, add just enough detail so that you know when you have arrived. Including *standards of measurement* will help you determine when you have achieved your vision of health.

If your vision includes "kind of, sort of, lowering my blood pressure," how will you know when you have arrived at your destination? "I want to have 120/80 blood pressure readings five days a week" is a very clear picture, with a clearly determined measurement.

"I want to weigh 10 pounds less" means you will never arrive at your destination; you will always want to weigh 10 pounds less than you do right now. "I want to weigh 135 pounds" is a clear, measurable goal.

Add time in your measurements as well. "I want to hike five 14,000-foot mountains *in the next year*" would require very different secondary choices than,

"I want to hike five 14,000-foot mountains *in the next 10 years*." You would take very different actions depending on the timeframe you chose.

When you have clarified your vision of health, write a description, including standards of measurement, in the section at the top of the chart.

4. Define current reality.

This fourth step differentiates this approach to creating health from all other "creating" strategies: *Where are you in relationship to your vision right now?*

Usually, this simple question is completely overlooked in any kind of goal-setting or visioning exercise, yet it is one of the most crucial. *If I don't know where I am, how can I begin to take effective action?*

Many "Law of Attraction" teachers encourage people to focus on their vision to the exclusion of what is happening right now. "Don't get bogged down with the details of where you are now! Just feel good and focus on that vision, vision, vision!"

Here's the rub, though. How can I know what step to take if I don't know where I am?

Imagine that I want to travel from San Francisco to Philadelphia, but I tell myself I'm in Chicago. How likely am I to make the correct decisions?

If you have no view of current reality, or no sense of where you are on the road, you are like a vehicle suspended in mid-air. Having a clear view of "current reality" —your current location in relationship to your vision—allows the rubber to hit the road. If you know where you are, you have *traction*. You have contact with the "road," in real time and can begin to make effective choices.

Your picture of current reality does not have to include everything in your life; instead, you need only the details that pertain to your vision. If your vision of optimal health includes weighing 135 pounds, for example, then current reality would include your weight *right now*.

Sometimes when I ask a patient to define current reality, she will say something like, "Oh, I usually weigh about 160 pounds."

"And what do you weight right now?" I'll ask again.

"Oh, a couple of weeks ago my weight really shot up, right after the family reunion and I really hate to say how much I weigh now."

Do yourself a favor: Get on the scale (if your vision includes weight). Write down exactly what the scale says, with today's date. If your vision includes maintaining a certain blood pressure, get out the blood pressure cuff and take a reading. Write down the results, noting the date.

Keep in mind that current reality will change over time. If weight is part of your vision and you are taking action, current reality *will* change. Accurately measuring current reality will allow you to assess whether or not your actions have been effective. For example, ask yourself: On my revised eating plan, have I lost or gained weight? How would I know if I hadn't accurately weighed myself to begin with?

5. Create structural tension.

You have created your vision of health, developed standards of measurement and accurately viewed current reality. The next step is to notice the difference between where you are and where you want to be.

In your mind's eye, imagine a big movie screen. Divide the screen in half, with a line running horizontally across the middle. In the upper half of the screen, create a picture of yourself in ideal health. In the lower half, create a picture of current reality.

If you want to weigh 140 pounds with 22-percent body fat, for example, see yourself in the upper picture stepping on the scale or reading your body composition machine with the results you desire. In the lower half of the picture, see yourself stepping on the scale and reading whatever your current weight is. Hold both of these pictures at the same time.

Usually, when you hold the two disparate pictures, you feel tension in your body. Robert Fritz refers to this as "structural tension." The disparity between where you are and where you want to be is like a stretched rubber band. The difference between vision and current reality is *potential energy.*

Think about how a stretched rubber band *snaps* when the tension is released. Usually, in the creative process, you continue to hold structural tension and utilize that energy over time to move forward, rather than releasing it in one dramatic snap.

Many patients are uncomfortable with the disparity between where they are and where they want to be. To relieve their discomfort, they do things to reduce structural tension.

The two primary ways you can reduce structural tension are to compromise your vision or misrepresent reality.

You may catch yourself saying things like, "Oh, I'd be happy if I weighed 155 pounds. I really don't need to weigh 135 pounds." In essence, you are diminishing your vision, bringing yourself closer to current reality. The rubber band has less "tension" when you downsize your vision.

You can also misrepresent reality by telling yourself you are closer to your vision than you actually are: "Well, I know I weighed 145 pounds last year at my annual physical. That was nine months ago, but I'm sure I'm still fairly close to that weight now."

Either method reduces structural tension, BUT it also eliminates the engine that drives you toward your goal. Lying about what I really want reduces tension, but it also diminishes the desire to create what matters most to me. Misrepresenting current reality means I am out of touch with where I truly am, in which case I probably won't make very good decisions.

Now, here's the great secret of working with structural tension: *Holding structural tension engages a whole series of unexpected means to achieve your vision.* The universe seems almost compelled to resolve the structural tension you create. You are naturally guided *to move along the path of least resistance.*

If you want to weigh 135 pounds, for example and know you need to exercise, you will be drawn to the form of exercise you most enjoy. Over time, as your body changes, you likely will choose different types of exercise. Water walking may be your first choice for exercise now. In a year, perhaps Jazzercise™ and yoga will be your cup of tea. In five years, Pilates™ and 5k marathons may top the list. Allow yourself to be drawn to the choices that are most appropriate *at this time*, knowing that they likely will change over time as you follow the path of least resistance.

Working with structural tension is an ongoing process, as both vision and current reality may change over time. "Optimal health" at 65 will probably look different than your vision of health at 25. Current reality will change over time as well.

Make structural tension your ally as it catalyzes your progressive movement from current reality to vision.

6. Choose your vision of health.

As you simultaneously hold your picture of health with the picture of current reality, ask yourself: "If I could have this picture of health, would I take it?"

This is an incredibly important question, because it truly *is* a question. None of us is *required* to be healthy!

Often, when I ask patients if they want to be healthy, they say, "Well, of course I do. Why else would I be here?"

Many, though, have come at someone else's urging, or they are interested in being healthy as long as it doesn't involve changing anything in their lives. They may initially choose their vision but then decide later that other things are more important than their vision of health.

Some common pitfalls to consider:

- I am choosing health to please my spouse/parents/children/friends (fill in the blank).
- I want to be healthy as long as I don't have to change anything.
- Sure, I want to be healthy, but I don't want to put any time or energy into my health. Can *you* make me healthy?
- I'm trying to implement someone else's definition of health.

You truly are free to say "yes" *or* "no" to your vision of health. I might envision sewing a dress, for example, and then later choose not to sew the dress. I may even have bought the fabric and pattern, but that does *not* mean that I am obligated to create the dress.

Answering the question "If I could have this picture of health, would I take it?" *honestly* is of central importance in creating your vision of health.

Choosing health is your *primary* choice. All of your other daily choices—e.g., what you eat or don't eat, whether or not you exercise, the way you communicate with people—are *secondary* choices that support your *primary* choice: to create your vision of health.

7. Make "secondary choices."

Many people pursue "health" by adopting someone else's idea of what health *should* look like and then follow one-size-fits-all recommendations. *Eight Weeks to Optimal Health* (Ballantine Books, 1998) by Andrew Weil, M.D., is an example of this approach. Although Dr. Weil offers many great suggestions, his ideas may or may not move you toward *your* vision of health. Your secondary, supporting choices will be tailored to your vision of health and your particular likes and dislikes.

Often, when you hold structural tension, secondary choices will occur to you. The woman wanting to weigh 135 pounds with 22 percent body fat, for example, might have the inspiration to call her friend Sallie who has been raving about a particular yoga class. She might also decide to eliminate the pat of butter that she spreads on her toast each morning (a study demonstrated that cutting out one pat of butter a day can result in a 10 pound weight loss over a year!).

You may also make secondary choices in collaboration with your family physician or other health care provider. If you want to begin an exercise program and suffer with severe heart disease, for example, you may choose to join a supervised exercise class, possibly in a hospital setting.

Your secondary choices will change over time, as you move farther from or closer to your vision. The woman pursuing her vision of weighing 135 pounds might start out in yoga class with her friend Sallie. Later she may discover she *really* loves swimming laps. Her exercise routine might shift to swimming three days a week and stretching with a yoga video at home twice a week.

When she reaches menopause, her weight program likely would shift again. Perhaps Pilates™ would be a better fit for her body at that time, or weight training with a personal coach in the gym.

Your secondary choices are likely to change over time. You may also begin a particular weight reduction program and discover that the diet has caused you to *gain* weight. You will need to choose a different dietary approach.

Remember that you have multiple ways of achieving your vision. You know what you want to create and you know your current location, but you do *not* know every single step of the journey (secondary choices). Even more importantly, you do not *need* to know every step of the way.

Consider the analogy of making a road trip from San Francisco to Philadelphia. You could take many different roads and even different types of transportation, to reach your destination. You might schedule a flight, ride a bike, or drive only "blue highways" on the map. Following any of these methods, you will arrive at your destination.

Avoid one-size-fits-all programs. Work with a health care provider who can help tailor a program to fulfill *your* vision and meet your particular needs and preferences.

Ideally, you would find a primary care physician who is familiar with many types of therapies and who can refer you to the most appropriate practitioners. Many health care providers who are trained in only one therapy or a narrow range of modalities are sure that their particular method will address all patients and all problems. Rarely is that the case. You likely will develop a team of health care providers to fulfill your particular vision of health.

If you would like more support in creating your vision of health, please visit *www.drjudithboice.com* for more information about The High Level Wellness Program©.

What to look for in a physician or other health care provider

With a clear vision of health, you can make decisions about the type of health care provider(s) you want to work with. The following questions can help you in that selection process:

- Does he offer you suggestions other than pills or surgery?
- Does she take time to answer questions?
- Is she interested in your vision of health? Although not necessary, sharing your vision of health can help guide your work together.
- How thorough is he in ordering tests to rule out possible diseases or conditions?
- Does the office return phone calls?
- Do you feel comfortable talking to your doctor? Are you able to express a full range of feelings and feel heard? Can you talk about "sensitive" subjects, knowing that you will be heard and the information will be held in confidence?
- Does your doctor aim to address the root of the problem, or just symptoms?
- Are you comfortable with your doctor's level of expertise?

This final question brings to mind a wonderful column someone posted on the message board in the clinic where I did my internship. The writer described her relationship with her "warm and fuzzy" family doctor, who for several years assured her that the lump on her breast "was probably nothing; let's just watch it for any changes." After five years of "watching" the lump, the patient pressed for more testing. The biopsy revealed a very aggressive form of cancer.

Over time, the patient came to appreciate her "geeky" oncologist, the one with the calculator in his breast pocket, who really knew his stuff about chemotherapy and radiation. "He didn't have the communication skills or the bedside manner my family physician did. But in the end, he saved my life," she concluded.

Great physicians combine "warm-fuzzy" communication skills with excellent medical knowledge. If you find a physician who combines people skills with medical knowledge, you have hit the jackpot! Sometimes you may find this combination spread over your relationship with several physicians; that is fine too. Appreciate the health care provider for the particular expertise he or she brings to the table. Ultimately, a combination of skilled providers creates an exceptional team, particularly if you are enduring a major medical crisis.

Abandoning the "doctor-god" model frees both you and the physician to develop a collaborative relationship. You both share responsibility in creating the level of health you desire. Working collaboratively opens the door for a completely different type of communication and interaction. Ultimately, *you* are responsible for your health care choices. Ideally, your physician would be your greatest cheerleader and your biggest fan in achieving your vision of health.

How can I find a qualified practitioner trained in natural medicine?

To help you find qualified "Green Medicine" providers, check the membership lists of the following national organizations. Although some very qualified natural medicine practitioners may not be members, these are reputable organizations to begin with.

Naturopathic *physicians*, for example, complete a four-year medical training and internship. In some states, naturopathic physicians are also required to complete a residency. In states that do not license naturopathic physicians, however, *anyone* can say she is a naturopathic "doctor." Colorado, the state where I live now, does not license naturopathic physicians. Sadly, we have had untrained, un-licensable "naturopathic doctors" misdiagnose and, in one case, even kill a patient. In an unlicensed state, a naturopathic doctor may have had a four-year medical training and maintain a license in another state; he may have completed a mail-order degree program, similar to a junior-college level of training; or she may have no training whatsoever.

The national organizations for naturopathic physicians and acupuncturists require practitioners to complete their training in an accredited school *and* pass national certification exams. Because the U.S. currently does not have any accredited programs for training herbalists, the American Herbalist Guild has a different method for certifying members.

Naturopathic physician

American Association of Naturopathic Physicians: *www.naturopathic.org*.

Licensed acupuncturist

National Council for the Certification of Acupuncturists & Oriental Medicine: *www.nccaom.org*

Herbalist

American Herbalist Guild: *www.americanherbalistguild.com*

Homeopath

www.homeopathicdirectory.com

Essential oil/aromatherapy practitioners

www.aromatherapycouncil.org

Flower Essence practitioners:

www.flowersociety.org

Bibliography for
The Green Medicine Chest®

Homeopathy

The Homeopathic Emergency Guide: A Quick Reference Handbook to Effective Homeo-pathic Care. Thomas Kruzel, N.D. 1993: North Atlantic Books.
Everybody's Guide to Homeopathic Medicines, 3rd edition. Stephen Cummings and Dana Ullman. 2004: Tarcher.

Advanced Homeopathy

Boericke's New Manual of Homeopathic Materia Medica with Repertory. William Boericke. 2008: B Jain Publishers.
Desktop Guide to Keynotes and Confirmatory Symptoms. Roger Morrison, M.D. 1993: Hahnemann Clinic Publishing.
*Repertory of the Homeopathic Materia Medica.*James Tyler Kent. 1990: B Jain Publishers.
The Science of Homeopathy. George Vithoulkas. 1985: Grove Press.
Organon of the Medical Art. Dr. Samuel Hahnemann. 1996: Birdcage Press.

Botanical medicine

A Modern Herbal: The Medicinal, Culinary, Cosmetic and Economic Properties, Cultivation and Folk-Lore of Herbs, Grasses, Fungi, Shrubs & Trees with Their Modern Scientific Uses. Mrs. Margaret Grieve. 1971: Dover Publications.
Herbal Medicine From the Heart of the Earth, 2nd edition. Sharol Tilgner, N.D. 2009: Wise Acre Press Inc.
Herbs in the Treatment of Children: Leading a Child to Health. Julian Scott and Teresa Barlow. 2003: Churchill Livingstone.

Holistic Herbal 4th Edition: A Safe and Practical Guide to Making and Using Herbal Remedies. David Hoffman. 2003: Thorsons.

Tom Brown's Guide to Wild and Edible Medicinal Plants. Tom Brown. 1986: Berkeley Books.

The Way of Herbs. Michael Tierra. 1998: Pocket Books.

Essential Oils

The Complete Book of Essential Oils & Aromatherapy. Valerie Ann Worwood. 1991: New World Library.

The Fragrant Mind: Aromatherapy for Personality, Mind, Mood and Emotion. Valerie Ann Worwood. 1996: New World Library.

Flower Essences

Australian Bush Flower Essences. Ian White. 1997: Findhorn Press.

The Bach Flower Remedies. Edward Bach and F.J. Wheeler. 1998: McGraw-Hill.

Flower Essence Repertory: A Comprehensive Guide to the Flower Essences researched by Dr. Edward Bach and by the Flower Essence Society. Patricia Kaminski and Richard Katz. 2004: Flower Essence Society.

The Healing Herbs of Edward Bach. Julian and Martine Barnard. 1988: Bach Educational Programme.

General Home Care

Acupressure's Potent Points: A guide to self-care for common ailments. Michael Reed Gach. 1990: Bantam Books.

Endangered Minds: Why Children Don't Think – And What We Can Do About It. Jane M. Healy, Ph.D. 1990: Simon Schuster Paperbacks.

Failure to Connect: How Computers Affect Our Children's Minds – and What We Can Do About It. Jane M. Healy, Ph.D. 1998: Simon & Schuster Paperbacks.

Home Remedies: Hydrotherapy, Massage, Charcoal and Other Simple Treatments. Agatha Thrash, M.D., and Calvin Thrash, M.D. 1981: New Lifestyle Publishing.

Parenting Well in a Media Age: Keeping Our Kids Human. Gloria DeGaetano. 2005: Personhood Press.

So Sexy So Soon: The New Sexualized Childhood and What Parents Can Do to Protect Their Kids. Diane E. Levin, Ph.D., and Jean Kilbourne, Ed.D. 2008: Ballantine Books.

Appendix

PREPARING FLOWER ESSENCES

Sun Method

- Begin gathering blossoms before 9 a.m. (dew still on the flowers) on a sunny day.
- Use a thin glass bowl, about 300 ml (8 oz) size, NOT oven-proof.
- Fill bowl with water, preferably spring water.
- Gather blossoms. Ideally, drop them immediately in the water-filled bowl. Have someone hold the bowl under the plant OR carry the blossoms on a large leaf and float them as soon as possible on the water.
- Even better, do not cut the flowers. Instead, build a platform to support the bowel so that the water reaches the flowers. This is the more ancient method of flower essence preparation.
- Place the bowl filled with water and flowers in the sun for 3-to-4 hours (less if the blossoms show signs of fading).
- No shadows, from you or grasses and plants, should shade the bowl.
- If a shadow falls on the bowl or clouds cover the sun, the remedy should be abandoned.
- Remove the flowers from the remedy using a twig of the plant, rather than your fingers.
- Notice how the water has changed!
- Pour the essence into a sterile bottle and add an equal amount of brandy, which preserves the essence.
- You can also pour the essence into a half-filled bottle of brandy.
- Label the bottle with the name of the essence.

Boiling method (most appropriate for thick, woody plants)

- Make the remedy on a clear, sunny day.
- Gather the flowers and twigs before 9 a.m.
- Fill a pan with spring water.
- Ideally, use an enameled pan; stainless steel is second choice. Do not use aluminum.
- As soon as you have gathered the blossoms, cover the pan and take it home.
- Cover the twigs and flowers with a quart of pure water.
- Place on the stove *without* a lid.
- Simmer for 30 minutes, using a twig of the plant to stir or press down the contents if necessary.
- After 30 minutes, remove the pan from the stove and carry it outside to cool.
- Remove the blossoms with a piece of the plant, not your fingers.
- Filter the essence.
- Place in a sterile bottle with an equal amount of brandy.
- Label the bottle.

Remember that you have made an *essence*. To make stock, place 2 drops of essence in 30 ml of brandy. To make medicine, place 2 drops of stock in 30 ml of water. *Eight ounces of essence will make millions of doses of medicine.* This is a very cost-effective form of medicine!

STUDIES ON THE CORRELATION BETWEEN COW'S MILK AND DIABETES

1   Dahl-Jorgensen K, Joner G, Hanssen KF. Relationship between cow's milk consumption and incidence of IDDM in childhood. *Diabetes Care.* 1991; 14:1081-1083.

2   Gerstein, HC. Cow's milk exposure and type I diabetes mellitus. *Diabetes Care.* 1993;17:13-19.

3   Work Group on Cow's Milk Protein and Diabetes Mellitus, Drash AL, Kramer MS, Swanson J, Udall JN Jr. Infant feeding practices and their possible relationship to the etiology of diabetes mellitus. *Pediatrics.* 1994;94:752-754.

4 Fava D, Leslie RDG, Pozzilli P. Relationship between diary product consumption and incidence of IDDM in childhood in Italy. *Diabetes Care.* 1994; 17:1488-1490.

WEB SITES

Flower Essences

Alaskan Essences: *www.alaskanessences.com*
Australian bush flower essences: *www.ausflowers.com.au*
Bach Flower Essences: *www.bachflower.com*
Flower Essence Society: *www.flowersociety.org*

Herbs

AmyLee, woodland medicine woman: *www.hernativeroots.com*
Gaia Herbs: *www.gaiaherbs.com*
Herb Pharm: *www.herb-pharm.com/*
Wise Woman Herbals: *www.wisewomanherbals.com*

Homeopathy

The National Center for Homeopathy: *www.homeopathic.org*

Naturopathic Medicine

The American Association of Naturopathic Physicians (four-year, medically trained): www.naturopathic.org

Essential Oils

Amrita Aromatherapy: *www.amrita.net*
Kurt Schnaubelt, Ph.D., blog on medical aromatherapy: *www.kurtschnaubelt.com*
Pacific Institute of Aromatherapy: *www.pacificinstituteofaromatherapy.com*

OTHER

Arise and Shine Cleanse: *www.ariseandshine.com*
Acupressure, with Michael Reed Gach, Ph.D.: *www.Acupressure.com*
The New Medicine Women: *www.medwom.com*

Author Biography

Dr. Judith Boice, award-winning author, international teacher, naturopathic physician and acupuncturist, is the author of several magazine articles and nine books, including *Menopause with Science and Soul: A guidebook for navigating the journey.* Dr. Boice graduated from the National College of Naturopathic Medicine, the oldest naturopathic medical school in the U.S. She has lived and traveled around the world, fostering an understanding and respect for many cultures and traditions.

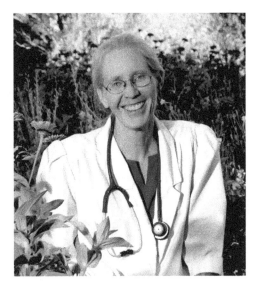

To contact Dr. Judith Boice for consultations or other information:

Web site: *www.drjudithboice.com*
E-mail: *drjudith@drjudithboice.com*

The Green Medicine Chest®

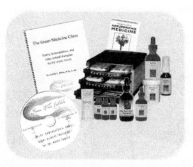

The Green Medicine Chest® brings together natural remedies with the knowledge to use them.

The Green Medicine Chest® introduces natural systems of health care through easily accessible video lessons and books, combined with a complete set of homeopathic and herbal remedies for use in your home.

The "Gold" version of the program includes:

- 4.5 hour training DVD
- Workbook
- *The Green Medicine Chest: Healthy Treasures for the Whole Family*
- Homeofamily Kit, with 33 homeopathic remedies
- 3 Essential Oils
- 1 Herbal Combination
- 4 Botanicals
- 1 Flower Essence
- Bonus: *"But My Doctor Never Told Me That!": Secrets for creating life-long health*

To purchase online visit: *http://www.drjudithboice.com/info/greenmedicinead4.html*

The Green Medicine Chest®: Healthy Treasures for the Whole Family DVD

This interactive 4.5 hour training provides the knowledge and practical skills to use:

- Homeopathic remedies
- Herbs
- Essential Oils
- Flower Essences

I had to write you immediately after I finished taking your course, The Green Medicine Chest®. What an amazing education you deliver in just two DVDs! This is by far the best source I have found for understanding how to apply natural medicine in my daily life. Thank you for further awakening my own natural healer and for teaching me how to respond to a wide range of illnesses and injuries by using "green" medicine.

KATHLEEN LUITEN
Medical Intuitive and Healer

For a preview of the DVD, and to order, visit:
http://www.drjudithboice.com/info/greenmedicinead4.html

Menopause with Science and Soul: A self-study program

This program, based on Dr. Boice's award-winning book *Menopause with Science and Soul: A guidebook for navigating the journey* provides you with information and encouragement to make this an exciting, transformative journey in your life. The program includes:

- *Menopause with Science and Soul: A guidebook for navigating the journey,* an exploration of the physical, mental, emotional, and spiritual changes that accompany menopause. The book explores the science of physical transformation, hormones, and biochemical changes during menopause. In addition, the book includes interviews with 14 women from different spiritual traditions, sharing their personal experience of menopause.
- Guided meditations from *Menopause with Science and Soul,* CD.
- "Menopause: A graceful change": a one-hour CD exploring five major lifestyle choices that influence our experience of menopause;
- "Celebrating Women: Sacred Chants for the Seasons of a Woman's Life," CD

- 12-lesson program that explores;

  - menopause as a normal, natural life passage
  - symptoms that can, but do not have to, accompany "the change"
  - hormones – what they do, and how their levels change as you transition through peri-menopause into menopause
  - how to decide if you are a candidate for hormone replacement therapy
  - the friendliest forms of hormone replacement
  - dietary factors that influence the menopausal passage
  - how exercise can strengthen bones and reduce menopausal symptoms
  - how to support bone health

To order, visit:

http://drjudithboice.3dcartstores.com/-Menopause-with-Science-and-Soul-A-self-study-program_p_50.html

High Level Wellness Program©

This five-week program guides you in developing a vision for your personal health and then making lifestyle choices that support you in fulfilling that vision.

What's included in the program:

- A copy of *"But My Doctor Never Told Me That!": Secrets for creating lifelong health* by award-winning author, Dr. Judith Boice
- Five 60-minute teleseminar classes
- A workbook to guide you through the program
- One 60 minute phone consultation with Dr. Judith Boice, to help guide you in developing your personal wellness program.
- The deluxe version includes three 60 minute phone consultations.

To sign up for the program, visit:

http://drjudithboice.3dcartstores.com/High-Level-Wellness-Program_p_57.html

Other Books by Dr Judith Boice

Menopause with Science and Soul: A guidebook for navigating the journey (Paperback)

Integrating modern medicine and ancient spiritual wisdom, *Menopause with science and Soul* is an intelligent and thoughtful companion to navigating the menopausal journey. Drawing from the latest medical studies, naturopathic physician Dr. Judith Boice advises women on practical concerns such as bone health, phytoestrogens, diet and exercise and, hormone replacement therapy, and offers stories, interviews, and rituals to nurture women's mental and emotional health. Essays and poetry from sixteen prominent writers celebrate the broad spectrum of women's menopausal experiences and honor diverse spiritual approaches to this significant life passage. Whether you're struggling with hot flashes or reveling in an unexpected rebirth of creativity, this comprehensive guide provides the scientific and soul-centered support you need.

To order, visit *http://www.drjudithboice.com/books.html*

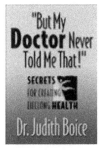

"But My Doctor Never Told Me That!": Secrets for creating lifelong health

Unveils the secrets for creating lifelong health, with step-by-step guidance to achieve your personal vision of optimal health. Instead of approaching health as a problem to solve, this book encourages you to create a vision of health, and then make lifestyle choices to achieve those goals.

After clarifying a personal vision, the book guides you through the foundations of nutrition, then exercise, and finally mental/emotional health. This information can be tailored with health care provider(s) to achieve individual health goals. Instead of short-term problem-solving, you will be on the road to making lifelong changes to benefit your health.

To order, visit *http://www.drjudithboice.com/books.html*

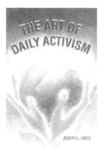

The Art of Daily Activism (Paperback)

The Art of Daily Activism is an invaluable guide to making the most of the politics of day-to-day life, combining the lessons of the mind, the heart, and a lifetime's experience. Envision a life worthy of your living and then create that vision in your daily life. "This book is for those who have dreamed, awakened to disillusionment, and remained determined to realize the stuff of dreams in the daily waking world. The heroes and heras are you and I, and our time is now."

To order, visit *http://www.drjudithboice.com/books.html*

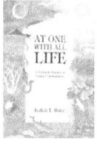

At One with All Life: A Personal Journey in Gaian Communities (Paperback)

At One with All Life is the story of Judith's life in four communities that shared a deep respect for the Earth. Judith lived at the Bear Tribe, a Native American Medicine Society; the *Findhorn Foundation* in Scotland; *Auroville* in India; and with traditional aboriginal people in Australia's Western Desert.

To order, visit *http://www.drjudithboice.com/books.html*

Index

BUY A SHARE OF THE FUTURE IN YOUR COMMUNITY

These certificates make great holiday, graduation and birthday gifts that can be personalized with the recipient's name. The cost of one S.H.A.R.E. or one square foot is $54.17. The personalized certificate is suitable for framing and will state the number of shares purchased and the amount of each share, as well as the recipient's name. The home that you participate in "building" will last for many years and will continue to grow in value.

Here is a sample SHARE certificate:

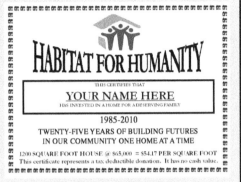

THIS CERTIFIES THAT

YOUR NAME HERE

HAS INVESTED IN A HOME FOR A DESERVING FAMILY

1985-2010
TWENTY-FIVE YEARS OF BUILDING FUTURES
IN OUR COMMUNITY ONE HOME AT A TIME

1200 SQUARE FOOT HOUSE @ $65,000 = $54.17 PER SQUARE FOOT
This certificate represents a tax deductible donation. It has no cash value.

YES, I WOULD LIKE TO HELP!

I support the work that Habitat for Humanity does and I want to be part of the excitement! As a donor, I will receive periodic updates on your construction activities but, more importantly, I know my gift will help a family in our community realize the dream of homeownership. **I would like to SHARE in your efforts against substandard housing in my community!** *(Please print below)*

PLEASE SEND ME _____ SHARES at $54.17 EACH = $ $_____

In Honor Of: _____

Occasion: (Circle One)   *HOLIDAY*   *BIRTHDAY*   *ANNIVERSARY*

     OTHER: _____

Address of Recipient: _____

Gift From: _____ *Donor Address:* _____

Donor Email: _____

I AM ENCLOSING A CHECK FOR $ $_____ PAYABLE TO HABITAT FOR HUMANITY OR PLEASE CHARGE MY VISA OR MASTERCARD *(CIRCLE ONE)*

Card Number _____ Expiration Date: _____

Name as it appears on Credit Card _____ Charge Amount $ _____

Signature _____

Billing Address _____

Telephone # Day _____ Eve _____

PLEASE NOTE: Your contribution is tax-deductible to the fullest extent allowed by law.
Habitat for Humanity • P.O. Box 1443 • Newport News, VA 23601 • 757-596-5553
www.HelpHabitatforHumanity.org